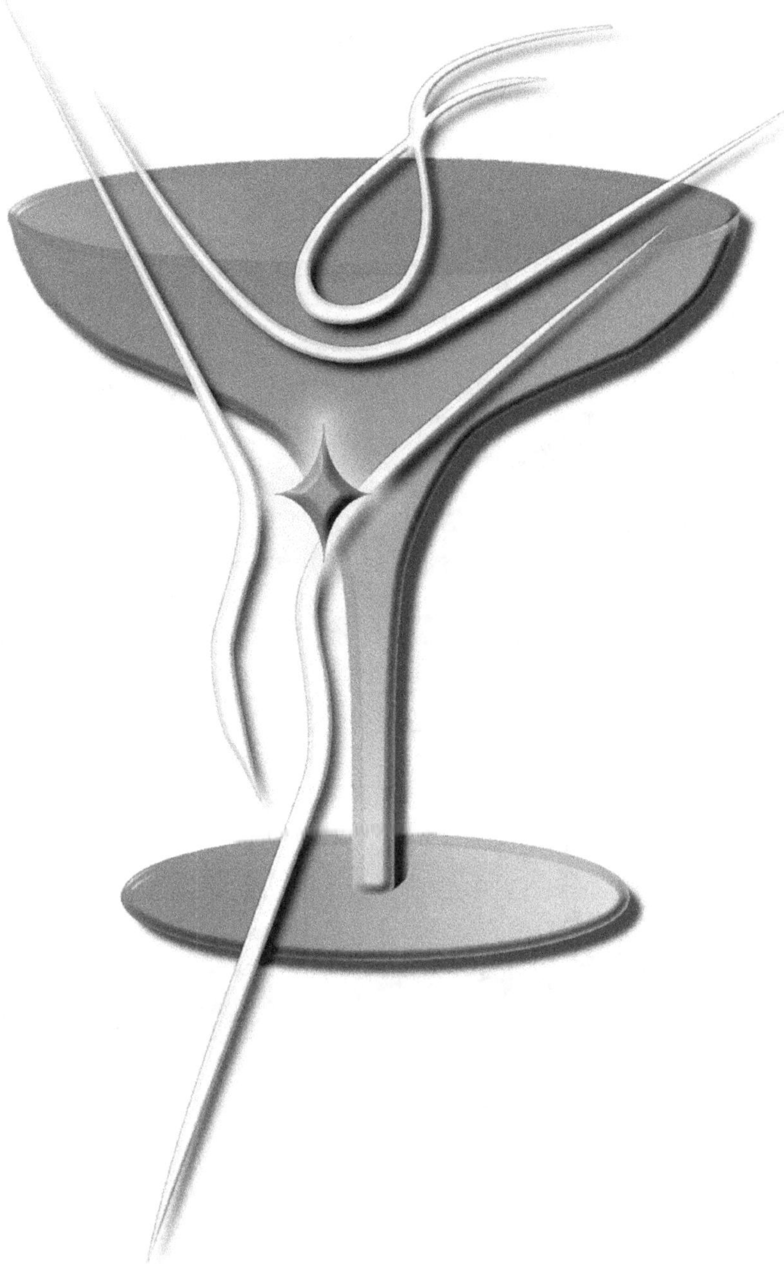

The "Pancreas Body Type"
is symbolized by a champagne glass.
Bubbly and joyful, they love socializing,
especially around food. With their genuine
concern for people and their ability to use
laughter to burst out of the most un-
comfortable situations, they bring
joy to their environment.

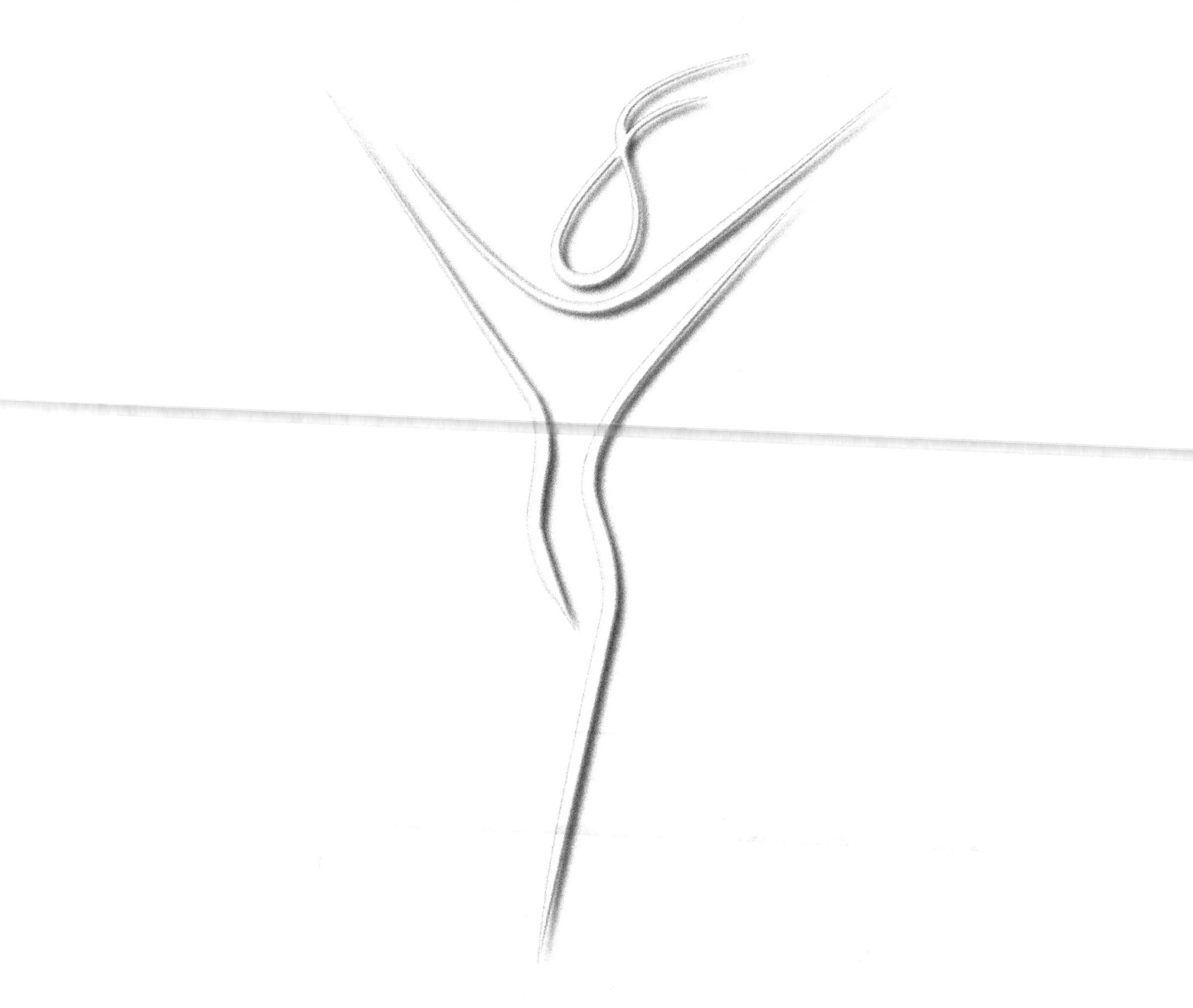

PANCREAS PROFILE & DIET

The Ideal Diet — *Does It Exist?*

An *ideal* diet is the one that nutritionally supports *your* specific dietary requirements. It's a way of eating that optimizes your health and vitality as well as normalizing your weight. Most diets are based on the myth that "One Diet Fits All." Many people think that if they can't stay on a diet, it's because they lack willpower. The reality is your body will have food cravings when it doesn't get the nutrients it needs.

The problem with most diets is that they are too general and do not address the specific needs of the individual such as "What time of day do I eat fruit or protein and which vegetables do I eat?" One diet does *not* fit all. Each person has a dominant gland, organ, or system that is stronger than the others which determines weight gain patterns, physical characteristics, and food cravings. This "dominant" gland is the basis of ***The 25 Body Type System***™.

Look to ***The 25 Body Type System***™ for the diet that truly supports your specific nutritional needs. Following your ideal diet will optimize your health and vitality as well as normalize your weight. Inability to maintain your ideal weight is the first sign of the body being out of balance. ***Different Bodies, Different Diets***™ gives you the dietary guidance to optimize your health.

Explanation of Terms and Format

Location & Function

Provides the location and function of the gland, organ, or system associated with each body type. The location is where, when healthy, the majority of the body's energy resides and, when depleted, where the body is most vulnerable.

Potential Health Problems

Identifies the problems your body type is prone to develop when your dominant gland becomes exhausted; includes early warning signs.

Recommended Exercise

Anaerobic exercise is essential for some body types, as it activates the immune system. Surprisingly, this isn't true for all body types. Some types are better with aerobic exercise such as yoga or Tai Chi since this type of exercise serves to rebuild the energy in the body. While exercise has many physical benefits, for most people, its greatest significance is in bringing about emotional well-being. Emotional benefits include releasing stress, clearing or calming the mind, and getting energy moving.

Exercise doesn't have to "look" like exercise. Ordinary daily activities can provide the needed movement required by some types. Included in this exercise section are the types of exercises that provide the greatest benefits.

One of the easiest ways to incorporate exercise is to use a fitness ball as a chair. Sitting on the ball forces you to use your pelvic and lower abdominal muscles. This improves posture and stimulates cerebral-spinal fluid movement, resulting in increased alertness and mental clarity.

Distinguishing Features

These features alone can often be sufficient to differentiate one body type from another. However, not every member of a type necessarily has them, or to the degree where they are strongly evident.

Additional Physical Characteristics

Supplementary characteristics are useful for comparing and contrasting different body types. Since physical characteristics reflect ethnic and familial heritage as well as dominant and sub-dominant gland characteristics, they can vary considerably. I've described the characteristics that are most commonly seen within each type and noted the ones that tend to run the entire range. For example, height in Liver types can vary from very petite to very tall, even though the majority is of average height. So, *don't rule out a type simply because one or two characteristics don't apply to you.*

Weight Gain Areas

Women: The initial weight gain pattern provides the most important—and often the simplest and most obvious criterion—for determining a woman's body type. Secondary gain refers to any weight gain over 15 pounds.

Men: Describes weight gain as to location and musculature appearance, including areas of primary and secondary weight gain.

Terms and Format

Scheduling Meals

A quick guide for choosing which foods to eat for breakfast, lunch, and dinner, and your ideal meal times.

Choose from the **Healthy** list when you feel strong and healthy, with plenty of energy available to digest your food.

Choose from the **Sensitive** list when your body is under stress (physical, mental or emotional). During these times, energy has been directed elsewhere and is less available for digestion.

Dietary Emphasis

Gives recommendations for weight loss or gain. Lists fat and protein requirements and their best sources. Fats supply essential fatty acids, but not all fats qualify to be included in the minimum fat requirement. Vegetarian diets support some body types, but not all.

Foods High in Amino Acids

Lists the highest sources that are most easily assimilated for your body type. The amino acids threonine, isoleucine and cystine are depleted when a person goes through a lot of changes or personal growth

Key Supports for System

Suggests foods and/or activities to optimally strengthen or support your particular body type.

Complementary Glandular Support

Identifies the two glands needing to be rebuilt or supported that will give your dominant gland a rest; suggests how this is best accomplished.

Foods Craved

(*When energy is low*) Lists the foods that, by stimulating the body's dominant gland, provide the greatest immediate, but temporary, energy lift.

Foods to Avoid

Identifies foods that are particularly difficult for your body to assimilate, or ones that cause excessive stress.

Recommended Cuisine

The cuisine most supportive to your system—particularly useful when you're dining out and need to select the most appropriate restaurant. Also included are the foods best suited to your type on a daily basis.

Psychological Profile

The Essence embodies the basic nature of each body type. The profile is often the deciding factor in body type identification. Relying on food preferences is often unreliable, since the desire for supporting foods can shift when the dominant gland becomes depleted. Psychological characteristics are often observed from birth and can be useful in identifying a child's body type.

Becoming familiar with the personality parameters of the various body types can help you gain insight into your own personal strengths and challenges, as well as expand your self-awareness. Additionally, aside from better understanding your own basic nature, increasing your knowledge

Terms and Format

Psychological Profile (cont.)

about the psychological dimensions of the other body types can enhance your understanding and acceptance of others different from you.

Greater awareness and understanding of yourself provides compassion and understanding of yourself and others. Being aware of the foods you eat and the effect they have on your body is often the first step in self-awareness.

Emotional Issues

While we all have all the emotional patterns, there are some issues that are more of a problem for some types than others. The emotional issues that create the greatest stress are the basic learning challenges for each body type and are listed here along with the other side of the emotion and the affirmation or way of shifting a negative emotional experience to a positive one.

Clearing an emotional pattern is achieved most quickly by connecting and releasing all aspects: the emotional, mental, physical and spiritual.

Feeling both sides of the emotion provides a focus and gives the blocked emotion a positive direction in which to move. Knowing both sides of the emotion allows for a mental understanding and brings the experience into a conscious awareness.

The spiritual aspect is achieved by the transition statement which provides a means of moving from the negative to the positive side of the emotion.

Essential oils access the limbic system of the brain which is the seat of emotion. When essential oils are applied to the alarm points, the cellular memory stored in the body is released.

To clear an emotion, smell the essential oil, feel both sides of the emotion, say the transition statement and apply the appropriate essential oil to the associated alarm point and the emotional release points on the frontal eminences of the forehead. Repeat as needed—whenever the emotion arises or you think about it, as well as at night before going to sleep.

More information is available in ***Releasing Emotional Patterns with Essential Oils,*** also by Carolyn Mein.

Visit ReleasingEmotionalPatterns.com

Physical Profile

Location	Left upper abdomen behind stomach, next to spleen and duodenum.
Function	Secretes enzymes that aid in digestion of proteins, carbohydrates, and fats; and secretes insulin, which helps to control carbohydrate (sugar) metabolism.
Potential Health Problems	Body utilizes or stores nearly everything consumed, and food generally high priority, so show strong tendency toward obesity (30 or more pounds overweight) throughout life. Frequently has family history of obesity, and possibly diabetes. Often has structural injuries due to weight (neck, shoulder, hip, ankle, foot pain). Tends to eat very rapidly; often emotional eater. Problems with digestion and proper utilization of fats and certain proteins. Vascular weakness, leading to fluid retention and headaches.
Recommended Exercise	Exercise is helpful, as it speeds up metabolism. Benefit is initially emotional. To maintain or reduce weight, exercising 6 days per week for 1 hour is required. Most effective times are morning or afternoon. Do exercises that are enjoyable, such as brisk walking, low impact aerobics, dancing, callanetics, biking, swimming, or hiking.

Women's Characteristics

Distinguishing Features	Tendency toward "rut" eating – eating same food 3 to 4 days in a row. Predominantly rounded appearance – particularly noticeable from behind in upper hips and buttocks. Small hands and often small feet, with little weight gain from knees to feet or elbows to hands. Known for bringing joy.
Additional Physical Characteristics	Buttocks rounded, with rounded upper hips. Excess fat initially firm, not flabby. Low back curvature straight-to-average. Breasts average-to-large. Shoulders narrower than, to relatively even with, hips. Waist defined to well-defined. Average to short-waisted. Height generally short-to-average. Bone structure small-to-medium. Average, elongated musculature. Hands generally small, unless large bone structure. Hair frequently thin or fine. Long rectangular, or average-to-long oval-shaped face.
Women's Weight Gain Areas	Lower body with initial gain in lower abdomen, upper hips, upper inner thighs, inner knees, middle back, and waist in firm rolls. Excess fat initially firm, not flabby. Secondary gain in entire abdomen, upper hips, entire back, upper arms, breasts, entire inner and possibly entire thighs extending to knees, buttocks, face, and under chin. Alternative secondary weight gain pattern: lower buttocks, lower hips and entire upper 2/3rds of thighs, outer thighs, extending throughout entire thighs – with cellulite predominantly on buttocks and thighs.

Physical Profile

Women's Weight Gain (con't)

Unless food intake is severely restricted, will gain weight easily when not exercising. Can put on large amounts of weight and have great difficulty losing and keeping it off. Often have suffered from weight problems most of life, with at least one overweight parent. May, however, have been thin earlier in life until having undergone period of stress.

Men's Characteristics

Distinguishing Features

Thick, straight torso with solid, prominent entire abdominal paunch. Soft layer of skin covering muscle, minimizing muscle definition across chest, back, and upper arms. Enjoy social activities, particularly when centered around food.

Additional Physical Characteristics

Buttocks can range from relatively flat to prominent. Low back curvature average-to-swayed. Shoulders relatively even with, to moderately broader than, hips. Solid musculature in torso with soft layer and entire abdominal paunch. Muscle definition in torso moderate-to-difficult to attain. Average-to-muscular thighs and calves. Height generally average to very tall. Bone structure medium-to-large. Hands can be small, or large when bone structure is large. Short, thick neck. Long rectangular or long-to-average oval-shaped face. Hair thin-to-average thickness. Hair-loss pattern is general thinning, frontal as rising forehead, or V-shaped point at center of forehead with marked receding at upper sides and may include back of head.

Men's Weight Gain Areas

Initial gain as soft thickening around waist, lower-to-entire abdominal paunch, often with soft layer covering torso, thickening in torso including chest, and under chin. Secondary gain as increased entire abdominal paunch covered by soft layer, soft or thick rolls around waist, marked thickening in torso and chest, hips, thighs, face, and under chin.

Dietary Guidelines

Scheduling "Healthy" Meals

Breakfast: Moderate, with grain, legumes, nuts, seeds, dairy, eggs, vegetables, and/or fruit.

Lunch: Heavy, with protein, legumes, nuts, seeds, dairy, vegetables, and/or grain.

Dinner: Moderate, early, with vegetables, protein, legumes, nuts, seeds, dairy, and/or grain.

"Sensitive" Meals

Avoid protein at breakfast and dinner. Fruit is recommended as evening snack only.

Dietary Emphasis

- Vegetables (mainly root type); complex carbohydrates, like rice, potatoes, beans, and popcorn; fruit, such as grapefruit, cherries, papaya, and pineapple; and protein, from such sources as fish or turkey (up to 10% of diet as dense protein) or, if vegetarian, from such sources as yogurt and cottage cheese. Rotation – ideally, 4-day, reduces pancreatic stress.

- For weight loss, caloric intake of 10-20% protein and 10-15% fat recommended. Will gain weight if fats fall below 10%. Rotate foods and vary them as much as possible; exercise for at least 1 hour 6 days per week; get ample emotional support; make lunch your main meal; avoid alcohol, caffeine, artificial sweeteners, and carbonated beverages; reduce salt, fats, breads, sugar, dairy, and quantity of food consumed; undertake detoxification program on seasonal basis; emphasize vegetables (particularly root); eat only at specified times; and employ variety. Consuming 10% dense protein helps maintain energy levels.

- Best to consume 60% of total food by 2 p.m. and, ideally, 100% by 7 p.m. Often easier to lose weight in summer than winter.

- For weight gain, eat regularly (avoid tendency to get so involved with something that you end up skipping meals).

- Vegetarian diet recommended for maintenance, since adequate protein can be obtained from vegetables and grains; although, may have up to 25% dense protein.

- Fats, 10-15% for weight loss, 25% for maintenance. Best sources are olive oil, nuts, seeds, butter, cheese, and dense protein (chicken, turkey, fish).

Dietary Guidelines

Foods High in Amino Acids
When going through a lot of changes or personal growth, the amino acids threonine, isoleucine, and cystine are depleted. They are highest and most easily assimilated in sesame seeds and tuna.

Key Support for System
Rotation of foods, as it reduces pancreatic stress. Eat recommended foods only at specified times; exercise; emotional support.

Complementary Glandular Support
Adrenals, through consuming dense protein (eggs, poultry, and fish), fruits, and vegetables. Liver, through emotional support (such as support groups – particularly helpful with weight loss).

Foods Craved
(When Energy is Low) Like most foods. Tend to crave same food (out of any food group) 3 to 4 days consecutively. Especially drawn toward sweets, such as chocolate chip cookies, peanut butter cookies and milk; creamy foods, such as ice cream; carbohydrates, especially potato chips, almonds, or mixed nuts; spicy foods.

Foods to Avoid
Alcohol, as it upsets blood sugar balance; caffeine, as it overloads kidneys; carbonated beverages, because they decrease oxygen in tissues resulting in fatigue; and artificial sweeteners, as they cause liver stress.

Recommended Cuisine
Chinese, Mongolian, Japanese, Middle Eastern, Moroccan, Thai, Italian, Mexican (delete the cheese); Soup and Salad bars.

Psychological Profile

Essence

Just as the pancreas, by breaking down carbohydrates or sugars, releases energy, Pancreas body types release energy, bringing joy. They love socializing, especially around food, and are usually the life of a party. Food, particularly sugar, produces energy. Likewise, Pancreases, in their exuberance, produce joy. Conscientious and reliable, when their energy is channeled into a particular area, Pancreases can be quite dynamic. They are the ones that continually release the energy that keeps an organization running. With their genuine concern for people and their ability to use laughter to burst out of the most uncomfortable situations, they are known for bringing joy to their environment.

Characteristic Traits

By nature, Pancreas types are highly sociable, caring, considerate, and compassionate. They tend to be able to maintain a certain joyous childlike quality that gives them a positive nature, full of laughter, joy, and lightness. With their delightful attitude, Pancreas types energetically transmit joy to those around them.

Food is a major issue for Pancreases and is connected with having fun. Since food is usually present in positive social experiences, it's easy for them to become "pleasure eaters." Going out to eat is generally the basis of getting together with friends. So when they're alone, Pancreas types tend to be "emotional eaters," using food to fill the void when they're feeling stressed, bored, or lonely. While Pancreases love to eat, they generally don't like to cook, so they tend to fall into a pattern of eating the same thing for several consecutive days. This "rut" eating stimulates their pancreas, but also depletes it. Consequently, it's very easy for them to put on excess weight, particularly when they've stopped a physically active lifestyle.

Pancreases like being with people, and enjoy bringing delight to their surroundings. Physically expressive, they like to touch, nurture, and help others. With an air of lightness about them, they are good at using humor to alleviate stressful circumstances. While the last thing they want to do is offend, being highly emotional, Pancreases are so enthusiastic that their spirited outbursts sometimes come across as pushy or overbearing.

Motivation

While Pancreas types are socially oriented and genuinely like people, they often experience problems in their relationships due to limitations in their communication skills. Focusing on accomplishing their agenda, they often comes across as being short or abrasive. Pancreases tend to need to talk a lot, to use others as sounding boards to sort through their thoughts and feelings in order to clarify them and get necessary feedback. This is usually stream-of-consciousness speaking, editing and refining as they talk aloud. Because of their inability to edit before they speak and in their haste to get the thoughts and feelings out, they may make a request sound more like an order or demand.

Psychological Profile

Motivation (*cont.*)

The tendency is to give orders, instead of asking, then to become hurt and upset when their interaction doesn't work. Being extremely zealous or emotionally excitable, they tend to speak about things with such animation and force that they come across as curt, manipulative, abrasive, or controlling. Then they can't understand why the other person seems upset or angry. Once they learn to communicate effectively, they're very considerate and caring of others.

The childlike trusting nature of Pancreases often sets them up for a rude awakening when someone they've put their faith in betrays their confidence. Because of their general innocence and lack of discernment, they may have difficulty evaluating the integrity of others, assuming honesty in another that's just not there. Not wanting to speak, act or express their own truth for fear of rejection or hurting someone else's feelings, truth and honesty become major issues. Unfortunately, when they are taken advantage of by others they believe in, Pancreases often experience deep hurt and disappointment that can cause them to close down and refuse to trust anyone.

Pancreases have a belief in lack and scarcity which is reflected in the way their body processes food. It will hang on to everything, getting the maximum benefit from every morsel. If the body is unable to process something it has taken in, it will store it as fat. This attitude of scarcity is reflected in the way Pancreas types need to have food around and keep their cupboards full. Because of the belief that there isn't enough, Pancreases take maximum advantage of every situation and store it up. They tend to hold on to things, getting locked into or attached to patterns, including eating the same food for 3 or 4 days, and resist change. Since food represents security, they often have a tendency to eat until their stomach hurts, especially as a child. Excess weight is a way of holding on to energy which represents security.

"At Worst"

Needy and insecure, Pancreas types will play the victim by living off anyone who will give them a handout, or staying in co-dependent relationships and getting locked into being a caretaker for someone else. In their desire for security in their relationships, they may neglect their own self-care. When they become overly stressed, they often withdraw into sleeping, burying themselves in a project, or go into hiding. Reluctant to make changes, they will set up and perpetuate a failure pattern, particularly when their significant initial effort was unsuccessful. Pancreases get locked into patterns of behavior that keep them from realizing the successes and fulfillment of desires that they seek. Feeling insecure is the same as feeling powerless.

There is often a fear of growing up, which may be associated with the fear of not being able to make it on their own. There is a feeling that too much is expected of them and a fear of not being successful. This is particularly true

Psychological Profile

"At Worst" (cont.)

when their initial attempts to excel or achieve have failed so further attempts to strike out on their own are often delayed due to a fear of repeating the past. Men often get caught in the Peter Pan syndrome of not wanting to grow up, wanting to stay in the safe spot of being taken care of forever. They will stay in co-dependent relationships until they evolve and find their truth, accepting themselves. The fear of stepping out on their own will often keep them in bad situations too long. The tendency is to internalize problems.

When insecurity levels are high, Pancreases generally have no sense of control, so they need to have boundaries and rules, particularly around food. They can easily become emotional eaters, putting on a lot of extra weight, particularly when there is insufficient joy or a feeling of insecurity. For men, the extra weight is often a way of saying, "I'm a big man and I have power." Their excess weight is generally an insulation for an inferiority complex due to not fully realizing or implementing what they know to be true. This inferiority complex is often instilled at an early age and the extra weight further instills it.

In areas where there have been past failures, the need for boundaries and rules is particularly high. Until Pancreases feel secure, they don't like grey areas, so they prefer to have everything black and white because it minimizes the chance of failure. They feel most comfortable when their jobs consist of tasks that are straightforward or well laid out for them. Projects that are ambiguous or overly complicated stir up feelings of inadequacy and fears of failure, bringing up past memories of personal defeat.

"At Best"

Highly sociable, Pancreases are at their best with others. Nothing gives them greater pleasure than bringing joy to their environment, which makes them extremely popular at social gatherings. Givers by nature, Pancreases are genuinely concerned with the welfare of others, and are among the most altruistic of the 25 body types.

Meticulous about learning new things, Pancreases take great pleasure in teaching others what they have learned. Often acquiring knowledge through experience, they can be quite resourceful when it comes to applying their newly discovered information. Enthusiastic and dependable, they work well with others and are good team players. Having a responsible and "take-charge" attitude, they will conscientiously see a project through from start to finish.

Loyal, steadfast, and dependable, Pancreases are good at routine or repetitive duties, successfully completing tasks that others may have abandoned as too tedious or hum-drum. They generally excel in areas where their work is well-defined. When a situation is clear-cut, they can apply new information and reliably complete the job.

Psychological Profile

"At Best" *(cont.)*

With a positive, vivacious nature, one that is full of laughter and lightness, Pancreases bring joy to everyone they're around. They love life and are interested in a lot of subjects, with their main focus being the people and their feelings.

Emotional Issues

Emotional issues that are basic lessons for the Pancreas body type are the fear of **betrayal**, fear of **letting go** and feeling **wrong**.

Betrayal is ultimately betrayal of self, although it is most often perceived as betrayal by someone else. The other side of betrayal is **trust**. The transitional statement is ***"I have the courage to accept the truth."*** The fear of betrayal is stored in the pancreas. The alarm point is located on the left side, below the breast in line with the nipple. The essential oil, **Forgiveness**, is used to release the fear of betrayal, apply to the pancreas alarm point and the emotional points on the frontal eminences.

The other side of *letting go* (fear of letting go) is **happiness**. The statement ***"Let go and let God"*** or ***"Let go and let live"*** provides the way to make the transition. Apply the essential oil, **Sage**, to the emotional points on the frontal eminences, and the bladder alarm point located in the middle, 3 inches above the pubic bone.

The other side of the feeling of *wrong* is **knowingness**. The transitional statement is ***"I am true to my source."*** The feeling of being wrong is stored in the accessory spleen located 2 inches above the lower edge of ribs, 1 inch from each side on front of body, right and left side. The essential oil, **Release**, is used to release the feeling of being wrong; apply to the accessory spleen alarm points and frontal eminences.

For a visual location of the alarm points see ***Releasing Emotional Patterns with Essential Oils***, also by Carolyn Mein.

Visit ReleasingEmotionalPatterns.com

Frequency Food Categories

The food lists are divided into 3 categories:

- *Ultra-Support or Frequently Food*s
- *Basic Support or Moderately Foods*
- *Stressful or Rarely Foods*

Frequency of foods refers to the individual food, rather than the entire group. For example, under grains you may eat semolina pasta twice a week, corn once as corn tortillas and once again as corn bread, and rye once as rye crackers and later as rye bread. This way you have your grains and variety.

Ultra-Support or Frequently foods are those that best support your particular body type and can be eaten most often—which means they can be included in three to seven meals per week. When you are hungry and can't think of anything that you especially want to eat, look at your *Frequently* list for ideas. Make sure you get variety from these foods, rather than relying exclusively on the same ones over and over again.

Basic Support or Moderately foods provide variety in your diet. These are the foods you would eat once or twice a week. The lists are designed to be as complete as possible, so don't let unfamiliar foods scare you. You don't have to eat something just because it's listed. However, since no single food contains all the vitamins, minerals, and amino acids, variety is essential. By adding the nutrients from different foods to your diet, you will provide your body with more complete nutrition than you would with a diet of limited food selections.

Stressful or Rarely foods are those that you should eat no more than once a month. While these foods aren't the best for you, the foods you seldom eat aren't usually the ones that cause problems, but rather those that you eat 80 percent of the time. So, being able to eat these *Rarely* foods once in a while eliminates the feeling of deprivation, especially if something you love happens to be on this list.

What happens if you frequently eat *Stressful foods*? They tax your body by taking more energy away than they provide. This is usually done through excessive stimulation of your dominant gland or overloading your digestive system. You will not necessarily experience an immediate stomach ache or headache after eating a stressful food. You could get a delayed reaction, ranging from mild to severe, that could include queasiness, upset stomach, mouth sores, lethargy, fatigue, constipation, diarrhea, dry or burning lips, dry skin, immune system weakness, nervousness, hyperactivity, or a craving for sweets. Symptoms may also be vague or hard to associate with a given food. Weight gain is often the result of eating too many of the *Stressful foods*, since the body will often store what it can't immediately assimilate.

By paying attention to what you are eating, you will eventually get to the point where you will be in tune with what your body needs. Once you are in tune with your body, you will have a good idea of what is best for you to eat or avoid at any given time.

As a small child you had an intuitive sense of what was right for you, as long as you had reasonable choices. At times, such as after a cleansing diet, you probably found it was easier to be aware of which foods you needed and which ones you shouldn't eat. Ideally, we want to recapture our childhood intuition and awareness of our body.

Since the body controls its own metabolic processes, it knows what it needs, and will be your best guide when it comes to what to eat. Your challenge is to correctly interpret the messages your body sends you. Generally, if you don't like a certain food, neither does your body.

Healthy vs. Sensitive Food Lists

Select foods from the *Healthy* food list when you feel strong and healthy. Select foods from the *Sensitive* food list if you have digestive problems, or when you are stressed.

The *Healthy* and *Sensitive* food lists constitute two parameters. Most people fall somewhere between them rather than being completely in one or the other. If you are basically healthy, start with the *Healthy* food list. As you look through it, you will probably find some foods you don't like or don't digest well. If these foods are in the *Ultra Support/Frequently* or *Basic Support/Moderately* category on the *Healthy* list, you will find they have probably been moved to the *Basic Support* or *Stressful* category on the *Sensitive* food list. Use the lists as a guide, being aware that the foods can change categories as your health or awareness changes.

The foods, food combinations, and menus are recommendations—suggestions designed to give you a place to start. Ultimately, you want to be aware of and listen to your body.

Menus: How to Select and Use

Often, menu selections in diet books include foods that don't work for certain people. Their systems might become overloaded by eating too many kinds of foods, or the foods are inappropriate for their body type. This could result in negative symptoms, such as a dull headache, mildly upset stomach, or lack of mental clarity. Another drawback is that the foods these menus recommend often take too much time to prepare. As busy as most of us are, cooking methods should be simple and uncomplicated. Cut down on preparation time by steaming, sautéing, or baking. Instead of rich sauces, season with herbs, combinations of herbs, or small amounts of salt and butter. Focus on menus that are practical. Once you have learned which foods are right for your body type, you can instantly evaluate any recipe as to how it is likely to affect you.

A wide range of menus have been included in this book, so if you run across a food, or food combination you simply cannot eat, cross it off and continue down the list. You are not limited to these menu suggestions, and as you work with the diet, you'll develop your own personal favorites. Quite often there are differences in food choices between types. What one person finds delicious may be downright inedible to another.

Each menu has been tested and approved by numerous members of the same body type. Not only are they tested for taste and desirability, but the food combinations are supportive for this particular type.

Food combinations are an important consideration, because a combination that is good for one type may not be good for another. It's not enough to simply eat protein with any vegetable. Knowing the combinations that are right for you allows you to optimize your diet.

For example, some types can combine almost any vegetable with chicken, while others need to be far more selective. Skin types can add broccoli, cauliflower, carrots, green beans, zucchini, asparagus, chard, mushrooms, or celery, using any one, **all** or any combinations. Thyroids, on the other hand, can combine broccoli and/or carrots, green beans, or asparagus with chicken, but not all of these at the same time.

You may wonder, is it best to eat your yogurt plain or add fruit? If you are a Pancreas body type, plain is best, but if you are a Pituitary or Kidney, add fruit.

Combinations can be responsible for how well you digest certain foods. Putting together the wrong foods can cause symptoms ranging from mild indigestion, a heavy or sluggish feeling, nausea, bloating, fatigue, irritability, and weight gain to stomachaches and allergic reactions.

Self-testing, or being muscle-tested by another person, can provide a valuable way to determine supportive food combinations. It enables you to determine what your body needs without interference from your conscious mind. Various food combinations can change test results, so when you are figuring out which foods your body really needs, keep asking until you find a combination that tests strong. Please remember that what your body wants today may be different from what it needs tomorrow.

Dietary Categories

Menus are categorized as *Healthy, Weight Loss, Weight Gain,* and *Sensitive.* The menu suggestions for losing weight are often the same as ones recommended for gaining weight, because achieving weight balance requires eating foods that best support your body. You may choose menus from various categories as your dietary requirements change.

Healthy includes all of the menus. It shows your potential, which foods you can eat when you are feeling well, and can be used for general body maintenance. Since it's the ideal diet for your type, it shows you how to get the best nutrition as well as how to combine foods that are especially appropriate for you. Different foods have been combined to complement each other. The criteria are:

1) A strong muscle response when testing them;
2) A positive physical effect after eating them.

Within a particular menu selection you will find food choices in parentheses. This designation means *with or without*—meaning these foods are optional and can be safely deleted from the combination.

Weight Loss menus are designed to be low fat and low calorie, paying particular attention to specific body type requirements. They often revolve around foods that help to detoxify the body, and include protein that is easily assimilated for rebuilding.

Weight Gain is for that neglected portion of the population rarely acknowledged as having a problem, specifically those who have difficulty maintaining adequate weight. People in this group are generally sensitive or have health problems interfering with assimilation. Also included here are athletes wanting to build muscle mass and people recovering from illness.

Sensitive menus are planned around the ***Sensitive*** food list. These foods provide the greatest support and are the most easily digested. Originally developed for people who had severely depleted their bodies or were extremely sensitive, these menus are to be used when you don't feel well, are recovering from an illness, or are under a lot of stress. If you find yourself in the ***Sensitive*** category, realize that as your system gets stronger, your foods will expand into the ***Healthy*** list.

Your body becomes extremely sensitive when it has been severely stressed—usually from chronic illness, prolonged fatigue, sleep deprivation, poor digestion or assimilation, hypoglycemia or low blood sugar, or as a result of obesity. This is when the sensitive diet is warranted. The basic sensitive diet, common to all the types, consists mostly of protein and vegetables. At times it will involve cutting down or eliminating sugars, including fruits, carbohydrates, and possibly reducing the grains down to only basmati rice.

One way to assist your carbohydrate metabolism is to give your pancreas a rest by restricting your carbohydrate and sugar consumption to a period of less than one hour a day. This allows the pancreas to secrete insulin only once, thus reducing stress on the body. Body types prone to pancreas exhaustion are the Pancreas and Skin types.

Some menus include ***Very Sensitive***, for people with extremely sensitive digestive systems.

The diets provided for the various body types are meant as a guide and can be modified to best suit your needs and desires. While your body is constantly adapting to changing conditions, the kind and quantity of food you choose to eat will vary with your activities.

Foods required to support your body during physical activity will differ from what is needed to support your brain during mental activity. Also, the amount of food you need at a particular time depends on what you are doing. If you are vigorously exercising, you will need to eat more than if you are sitting at a desk. The quantity of food eaten at meals will vary, as well as the choice of foods.

Example: Thyroid types can eat from almost any of the food groups during the day and in varying amounts, depending on how active they are. Those who expend a lot of mental energy during the day do best with a moderate breakfast of protein with a vegetable or grain, possibly followed by fruit juice or tea.

A mid-afternoon snack is desirable if you eat dinner late. The size and time of the evening meal often determines whether a heavy breakfast is wanted the next morning.

Regardless of your body type, it is important to change your diet appropriately when you are trying to heal, or when you are under stress. You should also adjust it if you increase your activity level, or if you change your environment.

Cleanse

A cleanse day is included with the one week sample menus to give your body a rest and chance to flush toxins. Cleanse duration can vary from one to three days, and you can change the frequency from weekly to every other week, or monthly, depending on your body and state of health. The menu itself will often include a variety of ways to prepare the food: steamed, raw and/or juiced. You can try any of the choices or vary them from week to week.

Ideally, on a Cleanse Day you give your body time to rest and pamper yourself. Just do what you feel like doing. It is helpful initially to visualize what you would like your life to be like five years from now—what you'll be like if you continue on the path you are on, and then see yourself making the changes you need to have the life you would like. This is also a good time to work on emotional issues associated with your body type.

Emotional Clearing

Each body type has certain core issues that are predominant. Even though we all have all the emotions, each body type has different lessons or challenges to work through. The core issue for your particular body type is listed at the end of the psychological profile. Another way to identify an emotional pattern is to read the "At Worst" section of the psychological profile. If you relate to a trait(s), refer to *Releasing Emotional Patterns with Essential Oils* for step-by-step instructions on clearing and releasing your core issues.

Relaxation Exercise

For a one minute relaxation that can be done as frequently as desired, close your eyes, relax your eyes and tongue. Focus your attention on your heart, see and feel a golden light coming from your heart and radiating out to all parts of your body.

If I follow the diet, what can I expect?

Stand before a full-length mirror in your underwear or a bathing suit. Turn and observe yourself from all angles: front, back, and side views. Take a careful look. Where do you appear to have excess weight? Do some areas look out of proportion, while others seem just right? Or maybe you need to put on a little weight in certain parts of your body?

The weight you carry on your body is a good reflection of how your system uses the food you eat. Eating the foods that are right for your particular body type and also observing the times of the day when these will be most effective for your system will enable you to give your body just what it needs.

This "conscious" eating will cause your body to lose unnecessary weight so that your system can function properly without the mental and physical stress of dieting. And, if you want to gain weight, it will be much easier as you will know what to eat as well as the times of the day when your system will get the best results from your food intake.

Eating for your body type is different from the usual weight loss diets, because now you are supplying your system with foods that truly support it. Weight loss diets usually stress deprivation of some kind, which often causes a rebound effect when you go off the diet. Eating the right foods for your body type allows you to reach and then maintain your correct body weight. This, in itself, is a step towards optimal health.

The most common comment I hear from patients who have begun to follow the diet for their body type, is "I feel better!" Many tell me that they have a higher energy level and that they no longer feel hungry between meals. Some are better able to avoid the sweets and caffeine that they were dependent on for that little boost they needed to get them through the day. Often they are able to accomplish much more because of better endurance, and they have more energy at the end of the day.

What it really comes down to is this: If you follow the eating regimen tailored to your particular body type, you will be using food the way nature, or your special nature, meant you to. When you support your body with a diet plan best suited for it, you can achieve an optimal state of physical health and well-being.

You must eat in order to live, so why not eat those foods that enliven you, unlocking the stores of energy and vitality that you may never have known before. And, with it, you can maintain that energy flow as it constantly replenishes and rebuilds your system.

Weight Loss Tips

Since gaining weight is often the first symptom of an imbalance in the body, the initial step to losing weight is to rebalance your body. The ***Healthy*** and ***Sensitive*** diets are designed to accomplish this goal. Occasionally, when people begin eating the foods they have deprived themselves of (sometimes for years), they put on weight. It's not uncommon to experience an increase in appetite for a short period before the system stabilizes.

There are a couple of pitfalls I'd like to caution you about. Some types have a strong tendency to ***go overboard on certain foods***, especially if they have been depriving themselves of them. If the foods happen to be high fat or high calorie, weight gain can result, particularly if the diet is not adjusted accordingly.

The next common problem is ***quantity of food***. The amount you eat is left to your discretion, as it will vary according to your activities and diet earlier in the day or week. Naturally, if you have been eating large meals, you may be ready for less food. However, if your food consumption has been low, your body may be needing more fuel.

Another cause of weight gain relates to ***muscle rebuilding***. When the body is robbed of adequate nutrients, it may consume muscle and replace it with fat. Later, this lost muscle must be replaced and fat eliminated. Dieters sometimes notice they weigh more after decreasing their fat intake and increasing their activity level. This is because all that rebuilt muscle weighs more than fat—so, it's best not to rely solely on the scale. Remember, fat takes up more room than muscle, so when you've lost fat, your clothes feel loose, even though your body weight may increase.

Generally speaking, two weeks on the *Healthy* diet is sufficient to provide the nutrients that may have been missing and to adequately support complementary systems, enabling the body to rebuild. Then the actual dieting can begin, employing the weight loss menus.

Emotional Eating

Are you overeating because you feel hollow inside? Do you use food, especially sweets, to reward yourself? Are these foods—particularly salty or fatty snacks—a necessary part of any social event? Do you nurture yourself with food? Do you use excess weight as a buffer? If you answered yes, and frequently, to any of these questions, you may want to check for an underlying emotional component. Negative emotions are fairly easy to recognize; fearing the negative consequences of expressing them, you might have a tendency to stuff these feelings, only to have them eventually surface. Since neither stuffing nor expressing negative feelings are viable options, you need a way to express them positively. The goal is to identify the positive emotion, access it, and express it.

All too often, even when we know the positive side of an emotion, we are so caught up in our negative programming we are unable to access it. Let's take anger for example: the positive side of anger is laughter. While laughter is a positive emotion, it can be surrounded by negative experiences. Therefore, being able to access the positive side of the emotion of anger as well as laughter requires clearing the negative energy around both.

Clearing an emotional pattern requires being able to access both sides of the emotion, understand the situation where it was created, learn its lesson, and then clear it out of cellular memory. Additional instructions for this process can be found in *Releasing Emotional Patterns with Essential Oils,* also by Carolyn Mein.

Conquering Food Cravings

Why is it that you sometimes have this awful, insatiable desire for a certain food at a particular time? Lemon meringue pie after a big meal, or a soft drink in the middle of the afternoon, or dill pickles when you are pregnant? What causes a craving, and how should you deal with it?

Food cravings usually involve your dominant gland and its need for stimulation. In order to overcome the craving, you need to understand what your body really wants. The urge to eat certain foods could be caused by emotional stress, or the need for specific nutrients missing from your diet. For example, the Thyroid body type craves sweets and carbohydrates because these are the foods that best stimulate the thyroid gland. When the body is stressed, the dominant gland—in this case, the thyroid—comes to the rescue and will continue to do so until exhausted and unable to respond. Once exhausted, symptoms of thyroid problems appear. In the meantime, the body craves foods that it knows will provide the greatest stimulation and the quickest energy lift.

Giving in to your food cravings will eventually cause you to overload your dominant gland, and put undue stress on your system. The way out of this dilemma is to understand why you crave a certain food and what your body is really saying with the craving. Basic nutritional needs are the basis for food cravings, so when you can determine what your system really needs, you can respond to this need in a way that supports your dominant gland as well as your body. Once you begin choosing the right foods in place of those that only stimulate, you are well on your way to achieving a healthy balance in your system.

Sugar Cravings

Craving sugar? (Sugar includes not only chocolate, candy or sweets, but also sweet fruit and carbohydrates like breads or muffins.) A desire for sugar is one of the first indications of protein deficiency. It's also common to crave sweets after eating too much protein. Since sugar is needed to get protein across the blood-brain barrier, a sugar craving could be your body's signal that you need to assimilate more protein.

Eating sugar, in any form, stimulates the thyroid gland, which controls metabolism. While you might feel more energetic immediately after eating sugar, its consumption leads to problems in the long run, because the underlying situation has not been properly addressed.

An energy drop, which often initiates sugar cravings, comes from adrenal insufficiency—often the result of fatigue or exhaustion. Rebuilding the adrenals requires protein and vitamin C. The protein most readily utilized is dense protein from sources like fish, chicken, turkey, and eggs, as opposed to vegetable protein like beans and other legumes. Broth-based soups are another easy way to assimilate dense protein.

Some people think they will benefit by increasing the amount of sweet fruits in their diet, citing their high vitamin C content. However, sweet fruit contains a lot of thyroid-stimulating fructose, which taxes the adrenals. Vegetables such as red bell peppers and broccoli can be better vitamin C alternatives. Focus on protein and vegetables for rebuilding the adrenals.

Artificial Sweeteners

You have been told you need to reduce your sugar and that refined sugar is bad because it robs the body of nutrients—so you think artificial sweeteners might be a good choice, right? *Wrong.*

The wood alcohol in the artificial sweetener, aspartame, converts to formaldehyde and then to formic acid, which in turn causes metabolic acidosis when its temperature exceeds 86 degrees Fahrenheit. Aspartame is marketed as Nutra Sweet®, Equal® and Spoonful®. In her lecture on aspartame, presented to the World Environmental Conference in 1997, Nancy Markle reported that methanol toxicity mimics multiple sclerosis, triggering systemic lupus and fibromyalgia symptoms. Some of the best sources of methanol toxicity are Diet Coke® and Diet Pepsi®.

Aspartame is not a diet product! The Congressional record said that it could make you crave carbohydrates and make you FAT. Dr. Roberts stated that when he got patients off aspartame, their average weight loss was 19 pounds per person. Formaldehyde stores in the fat cells, particularly in the hips and thighs. For web site addresses and more information on aspartame, check the *Resources*.

Food Assimilation and Weight Management

In order for a food to be considered a food, it has to contain fat, protein, and carbohydrates—even if the quantity is too small to appear on package labels. If any of these components are missing, the body doesn't register the substance as a food and won't assimilate it. Foods are classified based on their dominant component: fat, protein, or carbohydrate; e.g., meat is a protein, butter is a fat, and fruits, vegetables and grains are carbohydrates.

The assimilation of these foods, however, still depends upon the presence of all three components—fat, protein, and carbohydrates. Without them, digestion and assimilation are incomplete, which, of course, leads to a system imbalance.

Anything consumed that your body can't identify as being a food is considered toxic and treated accordingly. Too much of a toxic substance will overload the liver and may trigger a migraine headache or cause headaches in general. Sometimes the body will keep the toxic substance in fluid suspension, resulting in bloating or fluid retention. It may also be stored in fat cells.

Carbohydrates, which break down into sugar, are necessary for protein assimilation. This became quite evident when I began testing a product called Re-Vita®.

Re-Vita®

Re-Vita is a complete protein and contains all 22 amino acids. Initially, reading the ingredients, I was rather skeptical of its value, since the first ingredient listed was fructose (a sugar), and the main component was spirulina, an algae that few people are able to assimilate. Another ingredient was ginseng—an herb mostly considered beneficial for men, but not necessarily for women.

I was pleasantly surprised when I discovered that 70-80% of my patients, most of whom were very sensitive nutritionally, responded well to Re-Vita. I later learned that sugar was an essential factor in making this product easy to assimilate. Sugar enables protein to pass through a membrane between the bloodstream and the brain cells known as the blood/brain barrier. It also allows the same process to occur in other cells. So, Re-Vita duplicates what is naturally found in nature by using the fructose (sugar) to assimilate the protein (amino acids). This is also true for other sources of protein. It explains why carbohydrates are found in combination with protein in whole foods, and why we desire something sweet after a high protein meal.

Proper assimilation of food also requires the presence of vitamins and minerals, which are often deficient in processed foods. A vitamin and mineral supplement sometimes helps to provide these essentials, but knowing which supplements to use requires an understanding of the body's needs. Muscle testing is helpful in making the right selection.

Most vitamin companies manufacture a multiple vitamin/mineral supplement, but in more than twenty years of testing, I hadn't found one that was right for most people until I found Re-Vita. In addition to amino acids, Re-Vita contains vitamins, minerals, as well as trace minerals in a form that is easy to assimilate.

Most minerals are simply mined from the earth and put into capsules. Unfortunately, our bodies aren't designed to assimilate them in this form. Plants can convert minerals straight from the ground, but we can't. We can absorb them after the plants have converted them, or from animals who have digested the plants. If the plants don't absorb the minerals, they can't pass them on to us. This is why the algae used in Re-Vita is fed minerals, and why we assimilate minerals best from food sources.

Re-Vita is different in that the assimilation is made possible by feeding the minerals to spirulina rather than simply adding them to the formula. The algae then process the minerals into a form easily absorbed by the human body.

Food activates the digestive process. If vitamin pills are swallowed on an empty stomach, the stomach has no way of interpreting what's there. This is why the majority of nutritional supplements are most effective when taken with food. Consequently, mixing Re-Vita with food maximizes its effectiveness.

Popular Ways to Use Re-Vita®

*Use Revita in **Grains** as a:*

- sweetener on cereal like oatmeal, cream of rye or rice
- syrup on pancakes, waffles, or French toast
- flavoring for popcorn or in trail mix
- cookie—by melting butter, mixing oat flour, salt to taste, and Re-Vita, then adding fine cut raw oatmeal. Proportions vary depending on quantity and the consistency you prefer for your cookie. *(To make it stick together, forming a flat patty or ball, requires more butter. If you'd rather have it crumbly and eat it with a spoon, or use it as a topping over fruit or yogurt, use less butter.)*

*Use Revita in **Fruit** as a:*

- juice sweetener—add with water to unsweetened cranberry concentrate
- sweetener over cherries, rhubarb, or any other tart fruit. *(May also be used as the sweetener in fruit desserts)*
- lemonade—one lemon or two or three limes and one packet of Lemon/Lime Revita to one quart water (may drink exclusively for one to three days as a cleanse)

*Use Revita in **Dairy** as a:*

- sweetener and flavor for your favorite dairy product, such as yogurt, kefir, or milk (may add nuts, ie. pecans, pine nuts or almonds)
- coffee—adding 1/8 teaspoon of chocolate flavor to a cup of coffee will replace the nutrients depleted by the coffee

*On **Vegetables:***

- use Revita over squash or pumpkin

Basically, use Re-Vita as a sweetener on anything else that appeals to you. To obtain Re-Vita, see *Resources*.

Fats and Cholesterol

The body manufactures 70-90% of the cholesterol found in your blood stream. It uses cholesterol to manufacture hormones, antibodies and enzymes. Since enzymes are killed at 110°, cooked foods are enzyme deficient. To digest cooked food the body must then supply the needed enzymes. If the body is unable to digest what was eaten, it sends a signal to the liver to manufacture more cholesterol which is used to manufacture more enzymes. However, since the poorly digested food creates more stress on the body, the body often manufactures more hormones which it then stores as fat.

Hormones are manufactured in response to stress. Since the additional hormones are not exactly what the body needs, it stores them in the same regions it did during adolescence, i.e., as fat—leading to weight gain in specific regions, determined by your body type.

There is a lot of confusion around fats. Since fats contain more calories than protein and carbohydrates, many diets focus on the reduction of fats to reduce calories. Simply cutting out all fats or eating just any fat won't help, because you're not getting the essential fatty acids you need. This in turn triggers your body to produce more cholesterol, which leads to weight gain. Hormonal imbalances, such as hot flashes and mood swings, are often the result of a lack of essential fatty acids. Ideal sources for essential fatty acids your body can best utilize can be found under *Dietary Guidelines*.

Margarine vs. Butter

Butter is an excellent source of essential fatty acids, while margarine has been proven to have negative affects. Margarine is a product of hydrogenation, which produces trans fats—molecules that are harmful to the body's cell structure. These ***trans fatty acid compounds*** (TFA's) raise the levels of harmful cholesterol (LDL) and have been directly linked to increased risk of coronary disease, cancer and stroke.

Margarine is not the only source of trans fats. They are often found in breads, muffins, rolls, flour tortillas, breakfast cereals, cookies, peanut butter, chips and crackers. Trans fats are found in any product containing hydrogenated or partially hydrogenated oils. These products are often advertised as containing no cholesterol and include fake eggs, shortening, coffee creamers, and fried foods.

Heating liquid vegetable oils in the presence of metal catalysts and hydrogen produces trans fats. Processed food manufacturers and fast food makers prefer hydrogenated oils over unsaturated vegetable oils because they are solid at room temperature, have a longer shelf life and allow for high-temperature frying.

A comprehensive review of scientific evidence published in the June 24, 1999, issue of the *New England Journal of Medicine* confirms the connection between trans fats and coronary heart disease through their deleterious effects on cholesterol. Though trans fats do not contain cholesterol, they have an unhealthy effect on this substance once inside the body, raising the LDL, or "bad" cholesterol and lowering the "good" HDL cholesterol. This effect is essentially a double whammy for your arteries. Because these fats increase the bad while lowering the good cholesterol, it is estimated that the negative effect of eating them is about double that of saturated fats.

FAT: Total % of Fat Grams and Calories per Day

Total Calories per day	20%		25%		30%		35%		40%	
	Grams	Calories	Grams	Calories	grams	calories	grams	calories	grams	calories
1000	22	200	27	250	33	300	38	350	44	400
1500	33	300	41	375	50	450	58	525	66	600
1800	40	360	50	450	60	540	70	630	80	720
2000	44	400	56	500	67	600	77	700	88	800
2200	49	440	60	550	73	660	85	770	98	880

PROTEIN: Total % of Protein Grams and Calories per Day

Total Calories per day	20%		25%		30%		35%		40%	
	grams	calories	grams	calories	grams	calories	grams	calories	grams	calories
1000	50	200	62	250	75	300	87	350	100	400
1500	75	300	93	375	112	450	131	525	150	600
1800	90	360	112	450	135	540	157	630	180	720
2000	100	400	125	500	150	600	175	700	200	800
2200	110	440	137	550	165	660	192	770	220	880

How Much Fat and Protein?

Many diets emphasize low fat or low protein; as a result, I see many people who are fat and protein deficient. The average requirements I see are 25-30% fat and approximately 30% protein.

We have been told we need to reduce our food intake to 1000 to 1500 calories for weight loss. With weight being a chronic issue, I see many women who need to rebuild their bodies and initially require 1800 calories. Men generally require 2000 calories—and more if they do a lot of physical labor or exercise.

The table at the top of the page shows the number of calories and grams of fat based on percentage of calories from fats and the total number of calories consumed. The next table shows the same information for protein. On the following page are typical food examples with their gram and calorie content.

There are, however, some types, such as the Stomach body type, who need to reduce their fats to 20% to lose weight. Conversely, types like Gallbladder and Eye gain weight if their fat intake falls below 20-25%. Weight loss requirements can be quite specific, since not all fat sources are the same, and each body type has its specific sources from which to derive fat. This specific information is included in the *Dietary Guidelines Summary* section under *Fats*.

Fat, Protein and Calorie Content of Common Foods

FATS	Fat Grams	Protein Grams	Cal.
1 oz. almonds, dry roasted	14.7	4.6	167
1 med. avocado	30.8	4	324
1 oz. Brazil nuts	18.8	4.1	186
1 oz. Brie cheese	7.9	5.9	95
1 tsp. butter	3.8	<0.1	34
1 oz. cashews, dry roasted	13.2	4.4	163
1 oz. Cheddar cheese	9.4	7.1	114
1 oz. coconut, dry & unsweetened	18.3	2	187
1 oz. cottage cheese	1.3	3.5	29
1 oz. cream cheese	9.9	2.1	99
1 oz. feta cheese	6	4	75
1 oz. kefir, plain	1	1	19
1 oz. mozzarella, part skim milk	4.5	6.9	7
1 tbs. olive oil	14	0	120
1 tbs. peanut butter	7	4	90
1 oz. pumpkin seeds, roasted	12	9.4	148
1 oz. ricotta, part skim milk	2.2	3.2	39
1 oz. sesame seeds	14.1	5	162
1 oz. sunflower seeds	14.1	6.5	162
1 oz. Swiss cheese	7	8	100
1 oz. tahini sesame butter	14.5	5.1	169
8 oz. yogurt, plain, low fat	3.5	11.9	144

PROTEIN	Fat Grams	Protein Grams	Cal.
6 oz. fresh rainbow trout	7	45	257
6 oz. halibut	5	45	239
6 oz. haddock	2	41	190
6 oz. flat fish sole, flounder	3	41	200
6 oz. salmon	13	47	315
6 oz. shrimp	2	36	168
6 oz. light tuna packed in water	1	51	222
6 oz. roasted chicken dark meat, no skin	17	47	348
6 oz. roasted chicken breast meat, no skin	6	53	281
6 oz. roasted turkey dark meat, no skin	12	49	318
6 oz. roasted turkey white meat, no skin	6	51	277
6 oz. lamb chops lean, broiled	17	51	368
6 oz. center pork chops lean, broiled	18	54	393
6 oz. leg of lamb	13	48	326
6 oz. T-bone steak	36	42	507
6 oz. Porterhous steak	36	42	519
6 oz. roasted tenderloin	47	40	600
6 oz. round tip	30	44	467
6 oz. top sirloin	29	47	458
2 oz. 1 beef frankfurter	17	7	184
1 egg, large	5	6.3	75

Source: *The Corinne Netzer Encyclopedia of Food Values,* Corinne T. Netzer, N.Y.: Dell Books, 1992

Even though your diet may call for 25-35% of your total calories from protein, the amount of protein per day may vary. For example, you may be really hungry one day and eat more protein, maybe even 50%, then feel like eating only vegetables the next day. The recommended percentage is designed to give you a realistic guideline to be used as a dietary average. This gives you flexibility and allows you the freedom to ultimately learn to listen to your body.

To make sure you are getting the essential fatty acids you need, choose the majority of your fats from your best sources listed under *Fats* in the *Dietary Guidelines* section.

Snacks

For most body types, nuts and seeds are included among the best fat sources. Because they contain primarily fat and protein, nuts and seeds are excellent snacks. They provide quick energy and are easy to carry with you.

Roasted, unsalted nuts and seeds are usually easiest to digest and can be kept for extended periods of time in your car, purse, briefcase or desk. Unfortunately, the roasting process does kill enzymes. While eating them raw would be the best, most people have difficulty assimilating very many raw nuts and seeds unless they are soaked. Soaking activates the enzymes and helps remove acids, making them much easier to digest.

To soak, simply put some almonds, pumpkin or sunflower seeds in a bowl and cover with your drinking water. Let stand for 12 to 24 hours, then pour off the water (you can use it to water your plants). Take the quantity you want for the day and save the rest for later. Soaked nuts and seeds can begin to mold if stored at room temperature in a plastic bag for too long. However, they will keep for several days in your refrigerator.

Fruits

Dried fruit is easy to keep in your desk or carry in your purse. Taking fresh fruit and vegetables requires a little more forethought, but it's well worth the effort. Keeping your blood sugar levels up will keep you from grabbing a candy bar or overeating at the next meal.

Vegetables

Having trouble eating your vegetables, or getting your children to eat them? How old are they? If you are buying them from the supermarket, chances are it has been more than a week since they were picked. The life force in plants is highest when they are ready to be picked, not before. Once picked, they start to lose their life force or vital energy, so you want to eat above-ground vegetables within a week from the time they are picked, and ideally as soon after picking as possible. Root vegetables like potatoes hold energy longer. The greatest value of fresh food is its life force energy.

How fresh is your produce? When was it picked and how long has it been on the shelf or in your refrigerator? If your vegetables don't taste good to you and you are having difficulty eating them, check to see how fresh they really are.

Another cause of vitality loss in food is overcooking. What do you do if you can't get really fresh produce? Frozen vegetables often are the best alternative.

Amino Acids

The amino acids threonine, isoleucine and cystine are depleted when a person goes through a lot of changes or personal growth. The best sources are found in the *Dietary Guidelines* section.

Water

Our bodies are made up primarily of water. Consequently, the right kind of water in adequate quantities is essential. Approximately one-half gallon of water per day is ideal for most people. This sounds like a lot but it is only eight 8-ounce or four 16-ounce glasses. The Kidney body type often requires a little less, but most types need between 1-1/2 quarts and 3/4 gallon of water daily. If you live in a hot, dry climate or are especially active during the day, your requirements may increase.

Drinking water will curb your appetite. Many people eat, not because they are really hungry, but because they are dehydrated. In addition to flushing the toxins out of the body, water can help burn calories by metabolizing stored fat. Many people think that because a beverage contains water, it counts as water. Unfortunately, this is not true. The body registers liquids like coffee, fruit juice, soft drinks, soups, etc. as food. So, if you are drinking anything other than plain water, even though it contains water, the body can't use it as water.

The kind of water you drink will determine how easy it is for you to drink enough water. Heavily chlorinated water from the tap not only doesn't taste good but also adds toxic substances to your body. Since the main reason to drink water is to cleanse your system, drinking anything other than pure water is counter-productive. The best waters contain some minerals. This is why drinking water from a fresh mountain stream can taste so good. Distilled water leaches minerals, as can water filtered through reverse osmosis.

One way to upgrade water is to add a small amount of juice such as lemon, lime, apple, or grape. Sometimes this is enough to balance its mineral content and improve the taste. When you are dining in restaurants or traveling and must drink water from an unknown source, adding the juice of a lemon slice will help improve the taste and neutralize the chlorine, as well as other toxic substances. Adding a drop or two of peppermint oil will also upgrade water and aid digestion. Drinking peppermint water during air travel not only improves the taste of the water, but because it has anti-bacterial, anti-fungal and anti-viral properties, breathing the peppermint as you are drinking it can help protect you from air-borne microbes.

The best indication of whether a water is good for you is taste. If you don't like the taste of a particular water, it usually isn't the one that's right for you. It's easy to drink water when you like the taste. Muscle testing can also be used to determine your best water source.

Dietary Changes: "Take it Slow"

Listening to your body is being sensitive to your body's reactions to the foods you eat. This is important in making changes in your diet and also in starting special diets. Sudden changes in what you eat, even when you go from a poor diet to a healthful one, can produce negative effects in your system.

For example, when a person's system has deteriorated, whole, unrefined foods are usually indigestible. The body simply cannot tolerate a sudden change to a more healthful diet. A system that is used to highly refined junk food needs the fats and sugars that are easily metabolized for quick energy. These are stimulants that keep the system going but, at the same time, destroy health. If an individual is eating junk food, especially a child or a teenager, changing their diet should be done gradually. The body must be given time to adjust to new foods and eating patterns and to rebuild the weakened systems.

When foods can't be assimilated by an unbalanced system, switching to a healthful diet can leave the person devoid of energy. This alone could encourage one to abandon the diet and go back to unhealthy eating, which at least will supply the energy necessary to function.

So, before making any serious dietary changes, it is important to carefully consider what you are presently eating. Major changes usually need to be made in small steps, and care should be taken to eat those foods that will restore the depleted system.

Maintaining Your Diet

These diets are neither fads nor instant cures. It's about making permanent, long-term change. This lifetime eating program is based on sound dietary practices and what is individually right for each body type.

To get the greatest value out of your specific eating program, you'll need to change your eating patterns to the ways that truly support your body. In this process you will become more aware of when changes are necessary. Once you experience what it's like to feel really healthy, you will also know when your body is out of balance as well as how to regain that balance.

Long-term change rarely happens overnight, yet changing your eating habits can bring you better health and a more fulfilling lifestyle. Here's how some of my patients began to incorporate this program into their lifestyles:

> *"I looked at the diet, familiarized myself with what was ideal for me, and then compared it to what I was currently doing. I incorporated the parts that were easy for me, adding a single item I was attracted to, and put the diet away until I was ready for more."*

> *"I worked on one part at a time, first the foods, then the meals. The foods meant adding or deleting certain foods. Meals involved using new menus, mainly at breakfast."*

"I changed a pattern of eating sweets, like ice cream, cookies, candy, or pastries, from anytime during the day to only when my body could easily handle them. Now I save the sweets for later and if I still want them, eat them as an evening or bedtime snack."

"I shifted the time of day that I ate my largest meal from dinner to lunch time. It dramatically changed my energy level." (Pineal, Medulla, Skin, Pancreas, and Gallbladder types will definitely relate to this.)

"I followed the diet for 2 or 3 weeks and noted how I felt. Then I went back to the old way and noted the difference. I am convinced that it is definitely worth the effort to establish new patterns".

*"I added **balancing** foods. As a Medulla type, I found I could comfortably eat pepperoni pizza if I drank pineapple/coconut juice after it."*

"I started keeping a diary of what I ate and how I felt after each meal. I read my diary while I'm riding my stationary bicycle. This motivates me to stay with my diet and keeps me from sliding back into my old habits. When I first started following my diet a year ago, I felt great. Then I felt I was invincible and could eat anything. It worked for a while, but then I gradually started slipping back into my old habits. My headaches returned, my energy was down, and I became irritable and short-tempered. I went back on my diet and felt dramatically better. That's when I realized I needed to keep a diary to keep reminding me that I can feel great and what it takes to do it."

"Not everyone in my family is the same type..."

Rarely is every member of the family the same body type. Couples are often complementary types, sometimes opposites, and on occasion (usually with Pineals, Pituitaries, Stomachs, and Adrenals) the same. Perhaps one, and sometimes more than one child will be the same type as one of the parents. Most often body types in a family will be similar, and generally compatible—meaning that types corresponding to glands found in the head, such as the Pineal, are often attracted to similar types, such as the Thyroid, or to types whose dominant systems encompass the entire body, such as the Lymph, Blood, or Nervous System. To give additional examples, the Thalamus is quite compatible with the Hypothalamus, as is the Liver with the Kidney, Gallbladder, and Pancreas. Also, sometimes opposites will attract, such as the Pineal or Thymus being drawn to the Gonadal or Adrenal.

Returning, specifically, to type considerations as they involve family members, often the foods that can appropriately be eaten by one member will be similar to those acceptable for all members. As an example, let's say that in a particular family of five, all members can handle protein, grains, and vegetables for dinner—while two members can also have fruit. In this case, everyone could participate in the main meal, and the two who could handle fruit would have an additional option.

But what happens when the incompatible foods represent the main part of the meal—say, protein or grains? Balanced and Blood types, for example, do best when carbohydrates are the main emphasis for dinner, so pasta or rice with vegetables would be ideal. Those types who do well with more protein can easily add a protein entrée. A Pituitary woman, married to a Stomach man who needs substantial protein for dinner, can prepare a chicken dinner for the family, eat a light dinner herself (focusing, say, on vegetables and grains), and save her chicken for the next morning. This way, without having to cook two separate meals, she could get her large protein meal for breakfast, and still make it to work on time.

Assuming, however, that you're willing to change any former beliefs about family uniformity, you'll be ready to take the next step. To determine which meals are compatible for family members, check the food groups (protein, grains, vegetables, fruit, nuts, seeds, and dairy) that are the same, then compare the rarely foods for each type and eliminate them. Then you'll be able to plan your joint meals with this information in mind, adding additional entrees as needed for each family member.

Children and Diet

As a parent, you've probably experienced the frustration of having your child refuse to eat something, and not understand what was behind the refusal. Since children are in tune with their bodies (as we ourselves were before we programmed ourselves to ignore them), we need to respect their preferences yet at the same time not allow the child to control us through food. By knowing your child's body type, you know which is which.

Children are very sensitive to foods, and therefore greatly affected by what they eat. Many children will react to sugar, for example, which causes hyperactivity.

When glands, such as the adrenals, are stressed, the first response is hyperactivity; once depleted, they become exhausted. A child's system simply doesn't have the reserves of an adult, so selecting the appropriate foods for each meal becomes an important consideration. If you have a child whose body can't handle fruit in the morning, giving him orange juice will induce a sugar reaction that can look like hyperactivity and result in behavior problems. Or, if you have a child who requires protein for breakfast, not getting it can make him irritable, uncooperative, or hyperactive. There's also the question of what to give a child for a mid-morning snack. For some, fruit or fruit juice is ideal, for others, such a snack will trigger a sugar reaction. Some children are better off with carrot sticks, nuts or seeds; for others, an apple, or a combination of an apple with almond butter is perfect.

When it comes to overall health, what you eat as a child can make the difference between being a healthy adult and someone who suffers from chronic illness. If children are provided with a sound diet that supports their growing bodies, they can handle the dietary abuses of their teen years without succumbing to illnesses. These are the ones who grow up to be healthy adults less prone to illnesses and the effects of aging. Many of the chronically ill adults I work with suffered as children from earaches, headaches, colds, and flu, often having poor dietary choices available to them.

Microwave Cooking

The convenience of microwave cooking has overshadowed a number of studies that show it not to be the benign heating method it's assumed to be.

Microwave cooking is now known to alter the molecular structure of food, producing unhealthful effects. Studies done with breast milk, for example, show that warming it by microwaving causes a breakdown of proteins and antibodies, eliminating the natural infection fighting properties of the milk and destroying its ability to provide the passive immunity it would normally give an infant. This doesn't occur when conventional heating methods are used.

Other studies have shown that eating microwaved foods causes changes in blood chemistry similar to those present in the early stages of cancer. There's an increased tendency toward anemia, elevated cholesterol, and an immune response—as though the microwaved food is an infectious agent.

In addition to altering food molecules so they become difficult to digest or assimilate even under the best of conditions, microwaving destroys the enzymes that would aid in the digestive process. Although any form of cooking will destroy some enzymes, just two seconds of microwave energy destroys all the enzymes in a food.

Microwaved food causes the molecules to move so rapidly that they split in such a way that the body is unable to recognize them as food. The immune system responds to unrecognizable molecules in the same manner as bacteria and viruses, causing the immune system to work overtime. An overactive immune system results in allergies and autoimmune disease.

When food can't be digested fully, it becomes a toxic substance that must be eliminated, and the result is increased stress on the immune system. I often find that people experience a greater incidence of colds and symptoms of a weakened immune system when using a microwave oven.

Weight gain is also common. If the body doesn't have enough energy reserves to eliminate the toxins generated by eating microwaved food, it may gain weight as it stores those toxins in fat cells or suspends them in extracellular fluid. But not all body types react to toxicity in the same way. Some experience weight loss, especially if they normally have a hard time keeping weight on.

Individuals with very strong systems may not be aware of any adverse effects from eating microwaved food, as they are strong enough to absorb the energy drain without any obvious symptoms. However, the immune system is still under stress and will weaken over time. So it's best to avoid using a microwave for any food preparation, even defrosting foods or heating water. Avoiding microwaved food is vitally important for those who have weight problems or trouble with their digestive or immune systems.

Alternative Cooking Methods

I'm always amazed when I tell patients to give up microwave cooking at how many of them will ask me, *"If I don't use the microwave, how can I heat my food?"*

Go back to cooking the way you did before microwaving food became popular. *Steaming* is excellent, and if you don't want the extra moisture, use a *double boiler*. If you're heating food that contains a lot of juices, put it in a dish inside the steamer; this way the juices will stay in the dish.

When you're at work where you don't have a stove, use a portable *hot plate* or *fifth burner*. You can even bring your food in a corning ware dish so you don't have to wash an extra pan.

Toaster ovens are excellent for certain foods, as are *convection ovens*, especially if you want to reduce cooking time.

Leftovers can be heated in a ***skillet***, a ***frying pan***, a ***wok***, or by ***steaming***. When you cook, package the leftovers into individual serving sizes. This is a good way to get away from rut eating, because now when you're hungry you don't have to go to all the work of preparing a healthy meal. Simply take your food out of the freezer and put it in the steamer. This is usually what I do in the mornings for breakfast: I'll put something in the steamer, go take my shower, come back and it's ready.

Exercise Tips

Too busy to exercise? Here are some simple ways to incorporate exercise and body awareness into your daily activities.

Walking. To maintain proper body alignment and get the most out of your steps, focus on using the arch of your foot when you walk. Contact the ground initially with your heel, then roll on to the ball of your foot using the arch of your foot to lift your body. Simply focusing on the arches of your feet as you walk lifts your chest, aligns your spine, and puts a spring into your step.

Sitting. Does your seat get tired from sitting for long periods of time? Do you find yourself crossing your legs or sitting with one foot underneath you? This is your body's way of telling you it needs more space around your tailbone. The bones of your head actually move slightly every time you breathe, acting as a pump to move the cerebral spinal fluid (the fluid that coats the brain and spinal cord) down the spine. The sacrum and tailbone act as a pump to move the fluid back up again to the brain. When the sacrum is unable to move properly, the brain loses alertness and mental clarity. The answer is to sit so your spine can move by using a soft seat or sitting on a large exercise ball.

Using a ***fitness ball*** as a chair not only allows your sacrum to move, it improves posture, reduces wrist problems and strengthens pelvic muscles. The biggest cause of low back pain is lack of flexibility in the lumbar spine and abdominal muscle weakness. Simply sitting on the ball strengthens your pelvic and lower abdominal muscles as well as increases alertness and mental clarity. For additional information on the fitness ball, see *Resources*.

Healthy Food List

Healthy vs. Sensitive Food Lists	This is the *Healthy Food List*. For foods in the *Healthy Food List* that you don't like, don't digest well, or feel sluggish or bloated instead of energized after eating, move them down to a less frequent category. When you feel healthier, you may be able to eat them more often again.

Ultra Support or Frequently Foods
(3-7 meals per week—refers to each food rather than entire category)

Dense Protein Anchovy, catfish, cod, halibut, herring, mackerel, perch, red snapper, trout, water pack tuna; calamari (squid), crab, eel, lobster, octopus, scallops

Dairy Buttermilk, pineapple kefir, plain yogurt, butter

Cheese Feta, Jack, mozzarella, Muenster, Parmesan, low fat ricotta, Romano, Swiss

Nuts and Seeds Water chestnuts, almond milk, raw or roasted sesame seeds

Legumes Beans (garbanzo, great northern, pinto)

Grains Corn, corn tortillas, corn grits, corn bread, hominy grits, popcorn, brown or white basmati rice, Japanese rice, rice cakes, rye, durum wheat, pasta (all varieties), ramen noodles, bread (corn/rye, rye, pumpernickel, sesame pita bread), rye or sesame crackers, cream of rice, cream of rye

Vegetables Basil, cooked celery, corn, cucumbers, hominy, jicama, snow pea pods, potatoes (red, white rose), sweet potatoes, radishes, sea vegetables (dulse, kelp), squash (acorn, banana, butternut), raw tomatoes, yams

Fruits Apricots, cherries, grapefruits (red, white), guavas, papayas, nectarines, persimmons, pineapples (canned, sugar loaf)

Fruit Juices Apricot, cranberry, grape (purple, red, white), pineapple

Vegetable Oil Olive oil

Sweeteners Maple syrup, molasses, sorghum, honey, Re-Vita®, stevia

Condiments Sea salt w/kelp, ginger

Salad Dressing Dill salad dressing

Beverages Green tea; Calistoga® berry water

Healthy Food List

Basic Support or Moderately Foods
(1-2 meals per week—refers to each food rather than category)

Dense Protein

Beef, beef broth, beef liver, buffalo, lamb, veal, venison, organ meats (heart, brain); turkey, chicken, chicken broth, chicken livers, cornish hen, duck; ahi, abalone, sea bass, bonita, flounder, haddock, mahi mahi, orange roughy, salmon, sardines, thresher shark, sole, swordfish, yellowtail tuna; clams, imitation crab, mussels, oysters, shrimp; eggs

Dairy

Low fat or whole milk, raw milk, half & half, goat milk, sweet cream, sour cream, kefir (plain, peach, or strawberry), fruit flavored yogurt, ice cream (Dreyer's, Swensen's®), Ice Bean® (brown salt)

Cheese

American, blue, brie, Camembert, Cheddar, Colby, low fat or regular cottage cheese, cream, Edam, Gouda, goat, kefir, Limburger, regular ricotta, all yellow cheeses

Nuts and Seeds

Almonds, almond butter, Brazils, roasted cashews, raw cashews, cashew butter, cashew milk, coconut, filberts, hazelnuts, macadamias, macadamia butter, peanuts, peanut butter, pecans, pine nuts, pistachios, black or English walnuts, seeds (caraway, poppy, pumpkin, sunflower), sesame butter, sunflower seed butter

Legumes

Beans (adzuki, black, butter [lima], kidney, red, soy), lentils, black-eyed peas, split peas, soy milk, tofu, hummus, miso

Grains

Amaranth, barley, buckwheat, millet, oats, quinoa, rice (brown short or long grain, wild), rice bran, triticale, refined wheat flour, sprouted wheat, wheat germ, wheat bran, flour tortillas, cream of wheat, breads (Italian, French, oat, potato, sourdough, white), croissants, egg bagels, English muffins, couscous, macaroni, udon noodles, oat or saltine crackers, pita bread (plain, rye, or whole wheat), tabouli

Vegetables

Artichokes, arugula, asparagus, avocados, bamboo shoots, green beans, lima beans, yellow wax beans, beets, bok choy, broccoli, broccoflower, brussels sprouts, raw cabbage (green, napa, red), carrots, cauliflower, raw celery, chard, cilantro, eggplant, garlic, greens (beet, collard, mustard, turnip), kale, kohlrabi, leeks, lettuce (Boston, butter, endive, iceberg, red leaf, romaine), mushrooms, okra, olives (green, ripe), onions (chives, brown, green, red, vidalia, white), parsley, parsnips, peas, bell peppers (green, red, yellow), chili peppers, pimentos, potatoes (russet, yukon gold), pumpkin, daikon radishes, rutabaga, sauerkraut, sea vegetables (arame, nori, wakame), shallots, spinach, sprouts (alfalfa, clover, mung bean, radish, sunflower), squash (spaghetti, yellow [summer], zucchini), cooked tomatoes, turnips, watercress

Vegetable Juices

Carrot, carrot/celery, celery, parsley, spinach, tomato, V-8 ®

Fruits

Apples (Red and Golden Delicious, Granny Smith, Jonathan, McIntosh, Pippin, Rome Beauty), bananas, blackberries, blueberries, boysenberries,

Healthy Food List

Basic Support or Moderately Foods (cont.)

Fruits (cont.)   cranberries, gooseberries, raspberries, strawberries, frozen cherries, grapes (green, black, red), kiwi, kumquats, lemons, limes, loquats, mangos, melons (cantaloupe, honeydew, watermelon), oranges, peaches, pears, plums (black,   purple, red), pomegranates, rhubarb, tangelos, tangerines, dates, figs, prunes, raisins

Fruit Juices   Apple, apple cider, apple/apricot, black cherry, cherry, cranapple, grapefruit, guava, lemon, orange, papaya, pear, pineapple/coconut, prune, tangerine

Vegetable Oils   All-blend, almond, avocado, canola, corn, flaxseed, peanut, safflower, sesame, soy, sunflower

Sweeteners   Date sugar, raw sugar, refined cane sugar, brown rice syrup, barley malt syrup, corn syrup, succonant

Condiments   Dijon mustard, soy sauce, barbecue sauce, pesto sauce, salsa, tahini, horseradish, vinegar, eggless mayonnaise, soy margarine, Morton® salt substitute, sea salt

Salad Dressings   Marie's® Blue Cheese, Hain™ Creamy Italian, Hain™ Avocado, French, ranch, thousand island

Desserts   Custards, tapioca, puddings, chocolate, desserts containing chocolate, raspberry sherbet, orange sherbet

Chips   Bean, corn (blue, white, yellow), potato

Beverages   Raspberry tea, mint tea, herbal tea, black tea, Chinese oolong tea; mineral water, sparkling water; wine (red, white), beer, barley malt liquor, champagne, gin, liqueurs, Scotch, vodka, whiskey; regular sodas

Stressful or Rarely Foods

(No more than once a month)

Dense Protein   Pork, ham, sausage, bacon

Dairy   Nonfat frozen yogurt, most ice creams

Grains   Polished rice, whole wheat, cracked wheat, breads (7-grain, multi-grain, whole wheat), whole wheat crackers, whole wheat pasta

Fruits   Casaba or crenshaw melons

Sweeteners   Fructose, brown sugar, saccharin, aspartame, Equal®, NutraSweet®, Sweet'n Low®

Healthy Food List

Stressful or Rarely Foods *(cont.)*

Condiments   Catsup, yellow mustard, mayonnaise, margarine

Beverages   Coffee; Japanese tea; root beer, Pepsi®, diet sodas

---

Quick Reference Cards Provide a Convenient Format for Your Food Lists

Sensitive Food List

Healthy vs. Sensitive Food Lists	This is the *Sensitive Food List*. It contains all the same foods as the *Healthy Food List*. The difference is that when you are stressed or not digesting well, certain foods should be eaten less often. This list is the extreme – even when fairly stressed you should be able to eat most of these foods more often than stated. See how your body reacts to the foods and adjust accordingly.

Ultra Support or Frequently Foods
(3-7 meals per week—refers to each food rather than entire category)

Dense Protein   Water pack tuna

Dairy   Butter (sweet or light salt)

Nuts and Seeds   Water chestnuts, cashew butter, macadamia butter, sesame seeds (raw or roasted)

Legumes   Pinto beans

Grains   Corn, corn tortillas, corn bread, corn grits, popcorn, Japanese rice, rye, pasta (all varieties), ramen noodles, breads (corn, corn/rye, sesame pita, rye, pumpernickle), durum wheat, sesame crackers

Vegetables   Basil, cooked celery, potatoes (red, white rose), daikon radishes, squash (acorn, butternut), turnips

Fruits   Dates, raisins

Vegetable Oil   Extra virgin olive oil

Salad Dressings   Dill, Creamy Italian or Avocado

Beverages   Constant Comment® tea; Calistoga® berry water

Basic Support or Moderately Foods
(1-2 meals per week—refers to each food rather than category)

Dense Protein   Beef, beef broth, beef liver, buffalo, lamb, veal, organ meats (heart, brain); chicken, chicken livers, chicken broth, cornish hens, duck; abalone, anchovy, sea bass, cod, bonita, flounder, haddock, halibut, herring, mackerel, mahi- mahi, perch, orange roughy, salmon, sardines, shark, red snapper, sole, swordfish, trout, yellowtail tuna; calamari (squid), clams, crab, eel, lobster, mussels, octopus, oysters, scallops, shrimp; eggs

Dairy   Low fat or whole milk, raw milk, half & half, plain yogurt, Dannon® fruit flavored yogurt, pineapple kefir, Ice Bean®

Cheese   American, blue, brie, Camembert, Cheddar, Colby, low fat cottage, cream, Edam, feta, goat, Gouda, Jack, kefir, Limburger, mozzarella, Muenster, Parmesan, low fat ricotta, Romano, Swiss

Sensitive Food List

Basic Support or Moderately Foods (cont.)

Nuts and Seeds Brazils, coconut, filberts, hazelnuts, macadamias, peanut butter, pecans, pine nuts, pistachios, walnuts (black, English), pumpkin, caraway, poppy seeds, sesame seed butter

Legumes Beans (adzuki, black, butter [lima], garbanzo, great northern, kidney, red, soy), lentils, split peas, black-eyed peas, soy milk, tofu, hummus, miso

Grains Amaranth, barley, buckwheat, hominy grits, millet, oats, quinoa, white basmati rice, rice bran, rice cakes, white flour, wheat germ, wheat bran, white flour tortillas, triticale, breads (brown rice, French, Italian, potato, rye, sourdough, white), croissants, egg bagels, English muffins, macaroni, couscous, udon noodles, oat and rye crackers, cream of rice, cream of rye, cream of wheat

Vegetables Artichokes, asparagus, avocados, bamboo shoots, green beans, lima beans, yellow wax beans, beets, bok choy, broccoli, broccoflower, brussels sprouts, raw cabbage (green, napa, red), carrots, cauliflower, raw celery, chard, cilantro, corn, cucumbers, eggplant, garlic, greens (beet, collard, mustard, turnip), hominy, jicama, kale, kohlrabi, leeks, lettuce (Boston, butter, endive, red leaf, romaine), mushrooms, okra, onions (chives, brown, green, red, white, vidalia), parsley, parsnips, peas, snow pea pods, bell peppers (green, red, yellow), chili peppers, pimentos, yukon gold potatoes, pumpkin, radishes, rutabaga, sauerkraut, sea vegetables (arame, dulse, kelp, nori, wakame), shallots, spinach, sprouts (alfalfa, clover, mung bean, radish, sunflower), squash (spaghetti, yellow [summer], zucchini), sweet potatoes, yams

Vegetable Juices Carrot, celery, carrot/celery, parsley, spinach, tomato, V-8®

Fruits Apples (Golden and Red Delicious, Granny Smith, Jonathan, McIntosh, Pippin, Rome Beauty), apricots, bananas, blackberries, blueberries, boysenberries, cranberries, gooseberries, raspberries, strawberries, cherries, grapes (black, green, red), grapefruits (red, white), guavas, kiwi, lemons, limes, loquats, mangos, melons (cantaloupe, honeydew, watermelon), oranges, papayas, peaches, pears, persimmons, pineapples, plums (black, purple, red), pomegranates, rhubarb, tangerines, figs, prunes

Fruit Juices Apple, apple cider, apple/apricot, apricot, black cherry, cherry, cranberry, cranapple, grape (purple, red, white), grapefruit, guava, lemon, orange, papaya, pear, pineapple, pineapple/coconut, prune, tangerine

Vegetable Oils Olive

Sweeteners Honey, molasses, sorghum, date sugar, refined cane sugar, brown rice syrup, maple syrup, barley malt syrup, corn syrup, succonant

Condiments Black or white pepper, sea salt, chili pepper, tahini, salsa, vinegar, ginger

Salad Dressings Blue cheese, French

Beverages Mint tea, herbal tea, green tea, Chinese oolong tea; mineral water, sparkling water

Sensitive Food List

Stressful or Rarely Foods
(No more than once a month)

Dense Protein Pork, ham, bacon, sausage, turkey; catfish, thresher shark

Dairy Buttermilk, goat milk, cream, sour cream, kefir, nonfat milk, nonfat frozen yogurt, lemon yogurt, most ice creams

Nuts and Seeds Almonds, almond butter, cashews, peanuts, sunflower seeds, sunflower seed butter

Grains Rice (brown short or long grain, brown basmati, polished, wild), whole wheat, breads (whole wheat, sprouted wheat, 7-grain, multi-grain), saltine crackers, wheat thins

Vegetables Arugula, iceberg lettuce, olives (green, ripe), russet potatoes, banana squash, tomatoes, watercress

Fruits Casaba or crenshaw melons, nectarines, tangelos

Vegetable Oils Almond, all-blend, avocado, canola, corn, flaxseed, peanut, safflower, sesame, sunflower, soy

Sweeteners Fructose, brown sugar, raw sugar, saccharin, aspartame, Equal®, NutraSweet®, Sweet'n Low®

Condiments Soy margarine, margarine, catsup, mustard, mayonnaise, soy sauce, barbecue sauce, pesto sauce, horseradish, eggless mayonnaise, dijon mustard, Morton® salt substitute, baker's or brewer's yeast, ranch salad dressing

Desserts Custards, tapioca, raspberry sherbet, orange sherbet, chocolate, desserts containing chocolate

Chips Bean, corn (blue, white, yellow), potato

Beverages Coffee; sugar-free hot chocolate; black tea, Japanese tea; wine, beer, barley malt liquor, champagne, gin, Scotch, vodka, whisky; root beer, regular sodas, diet sodas, Pepsi®

General Dietary Guidelines

THE FOODS LISTED in the various categories are listed for natural, whole-healthy foods. Unfortunately, many foods in the United States have undergone changes that the human body is unable to recognize and process.

- The hybridized process increases *gluten* which stresses the digestive system.

- *Corn* has been genetically modified to kill insects that eat it by destroying the digestive system of the insect and thus, the insect.

Unfortunately, this process also damages the digestive system of animals and humans who eat them. If your digestive system is extremely strong and only a limited amounts of genetically modified products are eaten, you probably will not be aware of their effects. If your system is sensitive, you will want to avoid them.

What are Genetically Modified Organisms - GMOs?

GMOs are living organisms whose genetic material has been artificially manipulated in a laboratory through genetic engineering. This relatively new science creates unstable combinations of plant, animal, bacteria, and viral genes that do not occur in nature or through traditional cross-breeding methods.

What happened to wheat?

In the 1970's wheat underwent hybridization, and in the 1980's genetic modifications reduced its size which increased its yield and that was great for farmers. The changes made it possible for wheat to be used in other ways such as making pastries light, softer and easy to mold into different shapes. Producers realized that the new wheat strain was a potent appetite stimulant. That made it a big seller, and it took over the market place.

Soy is difficult to breakdown for most body types and is almost all GMO. It contains casein which is also found in dairy and difficult for many people to digest.

Dairy is pasteurized and also contains casein. If you are fortunate enough to have a good raw source, evaluate according to your body. Dairy, primarily milk and cheese, are often produced from cattle that have been fed GMO corn, so check your sources. Imported, aged cheeses, sheep or goat cheeses can be good choices. Butter and ghee are excellent fat sources that most people digest well. Kefir is a good probiotic source that can be used to re-establish the intestinal flora after the ingestion of antibiotics. It is possible to experience the effects of antibiotics if you eat commercially raised chicken or meat, like you would typically get when you eat out. Drinking 8 ounces of kefir over the course of 1 to 4 days, will re-establish the food source for the Candida Albicans to maintain a harmonious gut environment. Frequency varies, depending on your system and level of exposure.

General Dietary Guidelines

Sugar: Your intestines are covered with thousands of species of bacteria. The good bugs, or probiotics, work with your body to maintain good digestion. One of the ways the balance of good bugs and bad bugs can get thrown off is by eating too much sugar. When the gut's delicate ecosystem is thrown off, the bad bugs take over and this can result in many chronic illnesses and symptoms. Too much sugar in the diet may lead to diabetes, and is also responsible for a wide-range of health problems. These may include allergies, chronic inflammation, joint problems, digestive symptoms, mood and brain disorders, plus the growth of yeast. Too much yeast in the gut may cause chronic fatigue, loss of energy, general malaise, inability to concentrate, irritability, bloating and gas, frequent bladder infections, and other problems.

Sugar ideally should be limited to 6 tsp or 15 grams per day. This includes natural sugar that is found in fruit. One of the ways we inadvertently get a lot of sugar in our diets is in fruit juice, including smoothies. Dried fruit contains concentrated sugar, and even though it is good sugar, it is easy to mindlessly over-eat, so be aware.

How do I know if I could benefit from eliminating these foods from my diet?

If you suffer from inflammation and chronic pain, migraine headaches, digestive trouble including IBS, bloating, diarrhea or chronic constipation, thyroid issues, Autism, ADD or ADHD or allergies (there are 245 diseases currently associated with food allergies), you may want to start by eliminating the foods that produce the greatest amount of irritation for the greatest number of people. These foods are:

- *Sugar* — particularly refined, white sugar cane.

- *Gluten* — highest source is wheat. If you are extremely sensitive, you may want to start by eliminating all grains. White Basmati rice is the easiest grain to digest and a good place to start when you are reintroducing grains to your diet.

- *Corn* — Blue corn is often a good alternative as is organic popcorn

- *Soy* — almost all soy is now GMO, is hard to digest and contains casein.

- *Dairy* — except for butter - contains casein.

General Dietary Guidelines

If I eliminate all these foods, what am I going to eat?

Primarily **protein** and **vegetables**, along with **good fats**. However, even here you need to be aware. Common vegetables and fruit that are now GMO are zucchini, squash, alfalfa, sugarbeets and papaya.

While salmon is an excellent source of Omega 3 fats, you need to be aware that Atlantic salmon is not wild-caught, but farm-raised.

Fresh young **coconut water** is the closest food to mother's milk. It contains fat, protein, magnesium and acts as a digestive aid. Beware of boxed, canned or processed coconut water; there is a big difference between these and raw fresh young coconut in taste, quality and absorption. Many stores will open the young coconuts for you. Many tools are available online which make opening coconuts yourself easy. To store, pour the coconut water into a glass container with a lid, and add the soft coconut meat. If the meat is soft, you can scrape it out with a spoon. Coconut stores well in the refrigerator for 2 - 4 days or longer. Polarizing your refrigerator can extend the freshness up to 7 or 8 days.

Re-Vita® is spirulina that has been fed minerals, and contains all 22 amino acids. It was developed as an answer for world hunger to be added to milk, and in this combination, reverses symptoms of malnutrition in a few days. I like to add 1 - 2 packets of the Lemon/Lime flavor to the juice of a lemon or two limes into a quart jar and fill it with water. This is great during or after a workout, to sustain your energy throughout the day, a snack, or as a cleanse. During a cleanse, the Re-Vita lemonade can be drunk exclusively throughout the day, or used as a supplement. Re-Vita is sweet and is listed in the Food List under Sweeteners. Add it to oatmeal "cookies", mix it with almond or sunflower seed butter, or make a drink with the berry flavor, cranberry concentrate and water. Put it in your oatmeal along with nuts and butter; add it to butternut squash with cinnamon; or just put it in a spoon and swallow it when you are looking for something sweet to help you digest your meal.

Dietary Guidelines Summary

Focus

- Rotation of foods essential, ideally every 4 days to reduce pancreatic stress.
- Avoid dense protein for breakfast; minimize it at dinner
- Make lunch with protein your main meal between 12 and 2 P.M.
- Have an early dinner, between 5 and 7 P.M.
- Limit fruit to breakfast and morning and evening snacks.
- Emphasize protein and vegetables.

Dietary Emphasis

- From 25 to 35 percent of your calories are to come from fats.
- Best fat sources: olive oil, nuts, seeds, butter, cheese, and dense protein (chicken, turkey, and fish).
- From 20 to 35 percent of your calories are to come from protein.
- From 0 to 25 percent of your calories are to come from dense protein.
- Best sources of the three amino acids threonine, isoleucine, and cystine: sesame seeds and tuna.
- Caloric intake: 1,500 to 1,800 calories a day for women and 1,700 to 2,000 calories a day for men. If you are engaging in intense exercise (competition type) or hard labor, increase calories.
- Drink a minimum of 64 ounces of water a day. Drink water before and after meals, not with meals.
- Occasional desserts are best as an evening snack.
- Eat vegetables (mainly root type).
- Eat complex carbohydrates, like rice, potatoes, beans, and popcorn.
- Eat fruit, such as cherries, papayas, apples, and red grapefruit (with honey).
- Eat protein, particularly from fish and turkey or yogurt and cottage cheese.

Weight Loss

- Fat: 15 to 30 percent of daily calories.
- Weight gain will occur if fats fall below 10 percent of calories.
- Dense protein: 15 to 25 percent of daily calories.
- Rotate foods and vary them as much as possible.
- Exercise for at least 1 hour a day, 6 days a week.
- Get ample emotional support.
- Avoid bread, alcohol, caffeine, artificial sweeteners, and carbonated beverages.
- Reduce salt, sugar, and dairy.
- If you must have sweets, save for an evening snack.
- Reduce salt, sugar and dairy.
- Emphasize low-glycemic foods (e.g., sweet potato is OK but not white potato).
- Pay attention to your body regarding quantity of food: avoid overeating. Stop when satisfied.
- Best to consume 60 percent of total food by 2 P.M. and ideally, 100 percent by 7 P.M.

Dietary Guidelines Summary

Weight Gain
- Fat: 25 to 40 percent of daily calories.
- Dense protein: 15 to 25 percent of daily calories.
- Eat regularly (avoid tendency to get so involved with something that you end up skipping meals).

Vegetarian Diet

Recommended for maintenance, since adequate protein can be obtained from vegetables and grain; although, may have up to 25% dense protein.

Amino Acids

Best sources of the three amino acids threonine, isoleucine and cystine are sesame seeds and tuna.

Fats
- 10-15% for weight loss, 25% for maintenance.
- Best sources are olive oil, nuts, seeds, butter, cheese, and dense protein (chicken, turkey, fish).

Menu Key

These menus have been tested for ease of digestion and optimal nutritional support. The food combination consist of basic foods, allowing for complementary spices to be used to suit your taste. If desired, additional dishes may be included to enhance a meal. You will notice that some menu items are designated "**A**", "**L**", "**S**" & "**G**" *(see below)*. Some menu items are "L" or "G" while others have any one or a combination of designations.

"**A**" is for *adrenal rebuilding*. When the adrenal glands have become exhausted, the body needs additional support particularly at breakfast and lunch. The main adrenal rebuilding foods are protein and vegetables with limited fruit eaten at the specified time of day for your body type.

"**L**" is specifically for *weight loss*.

"**S**" is for *sensitive* and means this combination is very easy to digest and can be selected when you don't want to devote a lot of energy to digesting your meal, such as when you are fighting a cold or are under a lot of stress.

"**G**" is for *weight gain* or when you want to build extra muscle mass. Many times the menu is the same for both weight loss and weight gain because both much and too little weight are signs of the body being out of balance. The solution is the same—a diet that provides the nutrients you need to truly support your body.

When you are at your ideal weight you may choose from all of the menus. All menus may be used by healthy persons.

( ) around foods means these foods are *optional*.

Menus

A = *adrenal rebuilding*   **L** = *weight loss*
S = *sensitive*   **G** = *weight gain*   **()** = *optional*
(See previous page for more info on menu key)

BREAKFAST

8-9 a.m. Moderate, with grain, legumes, nuts, seeds, dairy, eggs, vegetables, and/or fruit.

SENSITIVE: *Avoid fruit.*

S Oatmeal w/Re-Vita®

G Oatmeal w/raisins, walnuts, or almonds, and plain nonfat yogurt

L Oatmeal w/banana

L Oatmeal, Rice Dream®, and strawberries

Cream of rice w/rice syrup, apricots, or cherries

S Cream of rice or cream of rye

Cream of rye w/Re-Vita®

S Cream of rye w/Amazaki™

S Corn grits or white basmati rice (small amount of butter)

L Grits w/berry Re-Vita®

S Couscous (butter)

S Millet in chicken broth

G Rice w/raisins, almonds, or walnuts, and plain yogurt

L Rice w/green peas or green beans

L Cream of wheat and pink grapefruit

Rice cakes w/sesame or almond butter, or sesame seeds

G Rice bread or rye toast, w/almond butter and banana

S Rice bread toast w/sesame butter or seeds

G Rye toast and raisins

L English muffin w/butter and apricot/pineapple jelly

L Plain bagel and pear w/cinnamon

S G Bagel w/cream cheese and Re-Vita®

L Raisin bread w/butter and cinnamon (pear or walnuts)

G Blueberry pancakes w/butter

Apple pancakes

Oatmeal/apple pancakes

G Pancakes w/Re-Vita® or jam

A L Poached eggs, rye bread, and grapefruit

A L S Eggs and mushrooms

G Scrambled eggs w/mushrooms and red peppers, cooked in olive oil, and pumpernickle bread

L Low fat yogurt w/Re-Vita®

L S Refried beans and corn tortilla

L S Baked acorn or butternut squash (butter)

L S Green peas (white basmati rice)

L S Yukon gold or purple potato, w/butter

L S Sweet potato (peas and/or butter)

L S Yam (butter)

Raw or roasted almonds w/apple

G Dried mangos, dates, or figs, and sunflower seeds

A L Pineapple and dry-roasted cashews or Brazil nuts

G Dates, nectarines, grapefruit, tangerines, or apples

L Re-Vita® or spirulina w/fruit juice and banana or pineapple

Blue/green algae w/apricot juice, banana, raspberries, or strawberries

L Papaya filled w/pineapple chunks

L Papaya, nectarines, tangerines, or apples

A L Papaya and raw sunflower seeds

L Dates, papaya, or strawberries

L Fresh peaches and sunflower seeds w/Body Trim tea

L Banana or mango and sunflower seeds

L Apple and raw or toasted almonds

L Pear and plain bagel w/cinnamon

L Grapes and almonds

L Red grapefruit w/almonds

L Pineapple juice

Menus

BREAKFAST OR DINNER

With meal.

L   Cranberry concentrate, berry Re-Vita®, and water

L   Good Earth® tea (Re-Vita®)

L   Apple sun tea – no honey

L   Red clover tea – no honey

L   Lemon mist tea – no honey

L   Raspberry patch tea

L   Chamomile tea

    Mint herbal tea

Note: *Use lemon juice in tea to neutralize acid.*

ANYTIME SNACK

Optional.

L   Wild berry zinger

L   Cafe Vienna

L   Orange cappuccino

MID-MORNING SNACK

(Optional) Grain, vegetables, nuts, seeds, protein, fruit.

L   California roll w/Bragg™ aminos

L   Trail mix

    Flour tortilla w/butter and orange spice herbal tea

S G   Fruit – such as dates, raisins, or pineapple

  G Papaya (pineapple)

L   Cranberry or raspberry Calistoga®

L   Mandarin orange spice tea or almond orange tea

LUNCH

12-2 p.m. Heavy, with protein, dairy, legumes, nuts, seeds, vegetables and/or grain.

A L G Sea bass or sole w/rice, carrots, and broccoli

A L S G Sea bass or sole w/white basmati rice or rice pilaf, and snow peas

A L S Sea bass or red snapper, white basmati rice, asparagus, or green beans

A L S Halibut or red snapper w/white basmati rice and yellow squash

A L Red snapper w/lemon, pepper and spinach

A L Mahi-mahi and stir-fry vegetables w/rice and low sodium soy sauce

A   G Broiled scallops w/butter, garlic, and green beans

A L Scallops, rice, carrots, and broccoli

A L S Tuna w/Top Ramen®

A S G Tuna w/noodles, zucchini, or green beans

A S Stir-fry: chicken breast, celery, onions, carrots, acorn squash, broccoli, and cauliflower

A L S Chicken sukiyaki

A L G Chicken teriyaki, basmati white rice, and butternut squash

A L G Chicken fajita, basmati rice, and steamed broccoli, cauliflower, and carrots

A S G Japanese spicy chicken and white basmati rice with tempura cabbage, broccoli, carrots, onions, and soy sauce

  S G Chicken and dumplings w/gravy

A L S Garlic chicken

A L Chicken, rice, and cole slaw

  L G Baked chicken w/Thai peanut sauce and vegetables

A S Chicken w/broccoli and carrots

A S Chicken (corn and/or red potatoes)

  L Turkey, cranberries, and carrots

  L Turkey sausage, brown rice, and green beans

    G Turkey, mashed potatoes, cranberry sauce, and gravy (peas)

    Beef and green beans

  S G Beef, red potato, and peas (onions)

  S G Monterey Jack cheese, alfalfa sprouts, and avocado on French bread

A L Eggs and potatoes (tossed salad)

Menus

LUNCH *(con't)*

L Stir-fry vegetables w/basmati rice and soy sauce

L Spinach w/Spike® and corn w/Bragg™ aminos

G Baked russet potatoes w/Monterey Jack cheese, and shredded cabbage and carrot salad w/creamy Italian dressing

L Hubbard squash w/butter and butternut Re-Vita®

L Lentils and brown rice

L G Red beans and rice

L Minestrone soup

S G Bagel, cream cheese, and Re-Vita®

L Hummus w/rice or sesame crackers

L G Carne asada burrito (rice)

S G Hummus, sunflower sprouts, and rye pita bread

L Bean and rice soup

MID-AFTERNOON SNACK

(Optional) 4 p.m. Grain, vegetables (no fruit for weight loss).

S Rice cakes

S Sesame crackers (butter)

G Squaw bread w/butter and butternut Re-Vita®

L S Popcorn

L Carrots, celery, or jicama

Salad: shrimp, cucumber, tomatoes, and red onion w/lime juice

S Fruit, such as strawberries or watermelon

L Mandarin orange spice, almond orange, or raspberry patch tea w/lemon juice

LUNCH OR DINNER

L G Mexican omelette

G Beef, white basmati rice, and spinach

L G Chicken burrito: flour tortilla, refried pinto beans, and salsa (rice)

G Turkey croissant sandwich w/turkey, lettuce, cheese, and avocado

L Turkey, rice, and cranberry sauce

A L Fish w/rice and corn, green beans, or peas

S G Pasta, mushrooms, and Parmesan cheese

L Pasta w/tuna and 1 Tbs Creamy Italian or 1/2 Tbs Poppy Seed Dressing

L Pasta and zucchini or green beans

L Noodles w/broccoli, carrots, peas, and onions

L S White basmati rice, broccoli, and butter

L S Broccoli and white basmati rice cooked in chicken broth

L S White basmati rice, butternut squash, and carrots, or peas

S Red, yellow, and green peppers sauteed w/onions and garlic over white rice

L S Sweet potato (butter)

L Mushrooms sauteed in butter and potato

L S G Pinto beans and white basmati rice, corn bread, or corn tortilla

L S Hummus w/rice cakes, carrots, and string beans

L G Baked falafel w/hummus and tomato (rye, or sesame pita)

L S G Split pea, black bean, or lentil soup w/corn muffin

DINNER

5-7 p.m. Early, moderate, with vegetables, protein, grain, legumes, nuts, seeds and/or dairy.

Sensitive: *Avoid protein.*

L Steamed potatoes, mushrooms, onions, and carrots

L Baked potato, butter, green beans, Spike®, and Bragg™ aminos

Boiled red potatoes w/butter and Vege-Sal®

Menus

DINNER *(con't)*

L		Butternut squash
L		Split pea soup and carrot salad w/creamy Italian dressing
L		Rice and steamed zucchini, onions, and dill weed
L	G	Steak w/steak sauce and broccoli or green beans
L	G	Barbecued chicken, peas, rice, butter, and Spike®
A L	G	Grilled chicken w/peas and yams
A L S		Chicken or chicken broth w/white basmati rice
L	G	Sushi (peas)
A L	G	Turkey or turkey ham, grits, butter, and black pepper
	G	Meat loaf w/tomato sauce, mushrooms, celery, onions, and peppers
A L		Tuna w/spinach and red onion
	G	Eggs, white cheese, and Italian bread
L		Hard-boiled egg w/rice cake, green beans, and Spike®
L S		Vegetable pasta w/butter
L		Pasta w/Romano cheese and sundried tomatoes (tomato sauce)
	G	Macaroni and cheese, and green beans
L S		Rice and steamed zucchini, onions, and dill weed
L		Spinach, avocado, and shrimp salad w/vinegar & oil, or Italian dressing
L		Caesar salad
	G	Spinach salad w/ creamy Italian dressing and cheese
S G		Pinto beans, white basmati rice, black olives, corn tortilla, and cucumber
L S		Sweet potatoes and cranberries
L S		Sleepy Time tea
L		Mandarin orange spice tea

EVENING SNACK

(Optional) 9 p.m.-2 a.m. Sweets, fruit, vegetables, nuts, seeds, grain, protein, dairy.

Note: *Only time when sweets, rich desserts or alcohol can be used in moderation with minimal negative effects.*

L	Watermelon or nectarine
	Orange juice
	Fruit, such as pineapples, dates, or raisins
S	Fruit, such as apples, tangerines, strawberries, or watermelon
S	Frozen cherries
	Lemon Sorbet
G	Ice cream (chocolate syrup, cherries, and/or macadamias)
G	Vanilla ice cream w/pineapple and cherries
G	Cookies and ice cream w/cherries
G	Honey roasted macadamia nuts
G	Raw pistachios
L	Sunflower seeds (raw carrot)
S	Seeds, such as pumpkin or sesame
S	Popcorn
S	Cookies
L	Toast and honey
S	Wheat Thins® or Keebler® Club Crackers
S	Sesame crackers (butter)
	Pretzels
G	Cheese streudel
G	Cherry pie and Sleepy Time tea
	Almond or lemon pound cake
	Protein drink

One Week Sample Menu

DAY 1 **BREAKFAST**
Oatmeal w/banana

LUNCH
Roast chicken & green beans

DINNER
Garlic shrimp w/pasta
(salad: Romaine, red, and green lettuce,
red cabbage, red onion, carrots, and
mushrooms w/balsamic vinegar)

DAY 2 **BREAKFAST**
Papaya or red grapefruit

LUNCH
Cod, sea bass or sole w/rice,
carrots and broccoli

DINNER
Caesar salad

DAY 3 **BREAKFAST**
Yukon gold potato w/butter

LUNCH
Roast turkey, corn, and cucumber

DINNER
Tuna (filet, canned or Japanese sashimi),
tomato (celery, lettuce)

DAY 4 **BREAKFAST**
Oatmeal w/sesame seeds

LUNCH
Beef or vegetarian chili w/avocado
and corn bread

DINNER
Pasta w/steamed zucchini & pesto sauce

DAY 5 **BREAKFAST**
Green beans, mushrooms and onions
w/white basmati rice

LUNCH
Halibut or red snapper w/lemon,
pepper & spinach

DINNER
Chicken livers w/beet salad

DAY 6 **BREAKFAST**
Banana

SNACK
Pumpkin seeds

LUNCH
Cornish game hen w/mashed rutabaga
& carrots

DINNER
Thai coconut milk soup or vegetable potato
soup and a tossed green salad

DAY 7 **BREAKFAST**
Yam w/peas (butter)

LUNCH
Scallops, sea bass or sole w/white basmati
rice or rice pilaf, and snow peas

DINNER
Corn tortilla w/refried beans & salsa

Alternative Menu Items

BREAKFAST

Refried beans & corn tortilla

Green peas w/white basmati rice

Corn grits or white basmati rice
(small amount of butter)

Cream of wheat and pink grapefruit

Eggs and mushrooms

Hummus and carrots

Pasta w/olive oil, zucchini, broccoli
and mushrooms

Baked acorn or butternut squash (butter)

Papaya filled w/pineapple chunks

Banana or mango and sunflower seeds

Sausage patty

LUNCH

Chicken fajita, basmati rice and
steamed broccoli, cauliflower & carrots

Baked chicken w/Thai peanut sauce
and vegetables

Turkey sausage, brown rice and green beans

Steak w/steak sauce and broccoli or
green beans or salad of butter lettuce,
celery, cucumbers, radishes w/dill salad
dressing

Pork chops and salad

Fish, rice, corn, and green beans or pea

Tuna, tomatoes and pickle

Bean burrito (salsa)

Rice bowl of chicken, broccoli, carrots,
onions, with soy sauce and ginger

Cobb salad w/eggs

DINNER

Noodles w/broccoli, carrots, peas and onions

White basmati rice, butternut squash,
and carrots, or peas

Pinto beans and white basmati rice,
corn bread or corn tortilla

Baked falafel w/hummus and tomato

Steamed potatoes, mushrooms,
onions and carrots

Grilled chicken w/peas and yams

Chicken and tomato

Sushi (peas)

Turkey or turkey ham, grits, butter
and black pepper

Tuna w/spinach and red onion

Feta cheese, cucumber, carrots, black olives,
hummus, and jicama w/olive oil

Sample Cleanse Menu

Ideally cleanse 1 to 3 days, 1 to 4 times per month

BREAKFAST

Watermelon or cantaloupe

LUNCH

Steamed cauliflower and/or squash and/or raw bell peppers, butter lettuce, carrots, celery and/or carrot/spinach juice

DINNER

Steamed asparagus, broccoli, and/or squash and/or raw carrots, jicama and/or juice of carrot, carrot/celery

Protein Powders and Supplements

When and how often to use protein powders, bars and food supplements with specific options for different times of day. Supplements are listed with most supportive first. Food items in parentheses () are optional.

ON RISING *(Choose one)*

NingXia Red™

Total Body Greens™

BREAKFAST *(Choose one)*

Pure Paleo Bone Broth™

Premier Plant Protein™

Lean Advantage™

Total Body Greens™

Premier Whey Protein™

Premier Nutritional Flakes™

Whole Body Collagen™

MID-MORNING SNACK *(Choose one)*

Pure Paleo Bone Broth™

Premier Plant Protein™

Re-Vita™ with cranberry concentrate, lemon or lime juice and water

NingXia Red™

Lean Advantage™

Total Body Greens™

Premier Whey Protein™

Premier Nutritional Flakes™

Whole Body Collagen™

Phyotein™

LUNCH

Natural food

MID-AFTERNOON SNACK *(Choose one)*

NingXia Red™

Total Body Greens™

Re-Vita™ with cranberry concentrate, lemon or lime juice and water

Premier Nutritional Flakes™

Whole Body Collagen™

DINNER *(Choose one)*

Pure Paleo Bone Broth™

Premier Plant Protein™

Balance Complete™

Premier Whey Protein™

Premier Nutritional Flakes™

Whole Body Collagen™

Total Body Greens™

Phyotein™

Lean Advantage™

EVENING SNACK *(Choose one)*

Designs for Health Protein Bar™

Re-Vita™ with cranberry concentrate, lemon or lime juice and water

Premier Nutritional Flakes™

Whole Body Collagen™

Total Body Greens™

Protein Powders and Supplements

NUTRITIONAL SUPPORT

(maximum weekly servings per supplement)

Young Living Essential Oils

(See your Young Living representative for these supplements):

Balance Complete™ - 2 times weekly

NingXia Red™ - 3 times weekly

Body Type Store

(Scan the QR code below for these supplements):

Designs for Health Protein Bar™ - 4 times weekly

Lean Advantage™ - 2 times weekly

Phytotein™ - 2 times weekly

Premier Nutritional Flakes™ - 7 times weekly

Premier Plant Protein™ - 2 times weekly

Premier Whey Protein™ - 2 times weekly

Pure Paleo Bone Broth™ - 5 times weekly

Re-Vita™ - may use daily

Total Body Greens™ - 5 times weekly

Whole Body Collagen™ - 7 times weekly

Visit BodyType.com.

Resources

PROTEIN POWDERS

Balance Complete™
by Young Living Essential Oils®

A daily nutrient and cleanse meal replacement containing 11 grams fiber, whey protein and Ningxia wolfberries.

Lean Advantage™
by Premier Research Labs®

Supports weight management, lean body mass and glycemic metabolism. World-class, full-spectrum ingredients include Green Coffee Bean Extract, Raspberry Ketones, and Citrus Aurantium extract – which helps promote fat breakdown.

Phytotein™
by Designs for Health®

Phytotein provides 20 grams of vegan plant-based protein and the amino acid lysine. This organic blend includes high quality non-GMO pea protein supplemented with sunflower, pumpkin seed, sacha inchi, and rice sources. A tasty and easily digestible alternative for those sensitive to dairy, gluten, whey, casein and soy. Available in chocolate and vanilla flavors.

Power Meal Vegan Meal Replacement™
by Young Living Essential Oils®

This nutrient-dense shake provides 20 grams of plant protein for powering through your day. 11 fruits and vegetables are enhanced with a dash of orange essential oil and vanilla. Rich in amino acids with zero added sugar. A balanced meal with fats, carbohydrates, protein and fiber, including 17 vitamins and minerals. Only 170 calories per serving.

Premier Nutritional Flakes™
by Premier Research Labs®

A quality source of vegan protein with a pleasant, cheesy taste. Non-GMO yeast provides bioavailable protein rich in B vitamins and amino acids. Sprinkle on salads, soups and other dishes for a hearty, cheesy taste. Only 40 calories per serving.

Premier Plant Protein™
by Premier Research Labs®

An organic, vegan protein powder including pea, which has been shown to subdue ghrelin, which sends hunger signals to the brain. Naturally free of allergens and ideal for those with food sensitivities. Provides 18 grams of protein. Supplies over 60 trace minerals without any synthetic ingredients.

Premier Whey Protein™
by Premier Research Labs®

Premier whey protein is a highly nutritious protein containing all 17 of the essential and non-essential amino acids. Premier's whey formula is guaranteed pesticide free, is produced using ultrafiltration at a very low temperature to preserve the broad array of protein molecules, including naturally occurring glycomacropeptides (GMPs) and is not toxic to the kidneys. It's great taste makes a wonderful smoothie or shake.

PurePaleo Bone Broth Protein™
by Designs for Health®

Contains a highly concentrated pure beef protein, produced through an exclusive hydrolysis and ultra filtration process. This process begins with beef from animals raised in Sweden, without hormones and free of any GMO grasses, grains, and ensilage. This purified beef protein contains both complete and collagen proteins that are naturally found in beef. Ideal for those who are dairy sensitive and want to build muscle, cartilage and ligaments from a true Paleo protein source. Comes in chocolate and vanilla flavors.

Resources

Pure Protein Complete™
by Young Living Essential Oils®

A whey-based protein drink designed to increase energy, strengthen the immune system, and build lean muscle mass. Flavors: Vanilla Spice and Chocolate.

Whole Body Collagen™
by Designs for Health®

Contains a unique blend of three patented collagen peptides supporting collagen production, bone strength, joint health and skin elasticity. Can be incorporated into shakes, smoothies, and other foods and beverages.

SUPER FOODS

NingXia Red™
by Young Living Essential Oils®

Made from Ningxia wolfberries. Provides dynamic energy and stamina without harmful stimulants. This anti-aging antioxident has the highest levels of ORAC activity. Supports the immune system, vision and liver. Visit **www.ningxiared.com** for information.

Re-Vita®
by Re-Vita®, Inc.

Spirulina that has been fed minerals and contains all 22 of the amino acids. May be used as a supplement or as a meal replacement once or twice a day. It comes in syrup form and is sweet. The average serving is 1 tablespoon.

Total Body Greens™
by World Health Mall™

An easy mixing, great tasting and energizing "phyto-nutrient" powder mix loaded with certified organic whole foods and plant extracts. Comes in original, berry, and chocolate with pure organic cocoa.

NUTRITIONAL BARS

Protein Bar™
by Designs for Health®

Small meal options, pre/post workout and be¬tween meal snacks. Optimal macronutrient blend for sustained energy and hunger control.

- *Bone Broth Chocolate Crunch Bar*
- *Cocommune Supplement Bar*
- *Peanut Butter Joint Power Protein Bar*
- *Yes Whey!! Ultimate Protein Bar*
- *Bold Beauty Collagen Protein Bar*
- *Plant-Powered Magnesium Protein Bar*

Resources

OTHER FOODS

Coconut Oil
By Tropical Traditions®

Coconut oil is one of the best cooking oils to use and is rich in lauric acid which supports the immune system. It is unrefined, organic, no trans fatty acids, and provides energy which can lead to weight loss.

Pink Salt
By Premier Research Labs®

Unrefined, untreated sea salt containing valuable trace elements not found in regular table salt.

VIBRATIONALS

Father Genetics & Mother Genetics

While in utero and during infancy, we pick up emotions, attitudes, and perspectives from our parents and their genetic lines that we collect and adopt as our own. Some of these we would like to keep, while many of these can be hindrances to where we want to be in life. Father Genetics and Mother Genetics bring to your awareness where these patterns come from and allow you to consciously decide if you want to keep them, adapt them, transmute them or simply release them.

PRODUCTS

EMF Neutralizer (for cellphones) – Puts a positive energy field around the phone, neutralizing potentially harmful radiation. May also be used on devices such as computers, portable phones, or digital watches.

Living Water House System – Makes water taste good, helps dry skin and helps hydration of cells. De-scales plumbing and enhances plant growth.

Living Water Pool Patch – Makes skin softer, decreases stinging eyes and fading clothes. Reduces scale build-up, making cleaning easier and makes equipment last longer.

Chakra Harmony DVD – This easy to follow DVD will show you how to balance your life energies and relieve stress. Can be used actively or as a soothing background for relaxing and revitalizing yourself and others. Suitable for all ages, combines visual and sound toning techniques to harmonize your body, mind and spirit.

Chakra Essential Oils Kit – Safety pack with eight Chakra Essential Oils. For added enhancement, combine the Chakra Harmony DVD with the eight recommended Essential Chakra Oils to further your awareness of your healing senses.

EXERCISE

Fitness Ball – The easiest way to exercise. Incorporate exercise into your lifestyle by using a fitness ball as a chair. The weakest point of the body is the pelvis which results in weakness of the lower abdominal muscles and low back pain. Sitting on the ball forces you to use your pelvic and lower abdominal muscles. This improves posture, reduces wrist problems, and stimulates cerebral-spinal fluid movement, resulting in increased alertness and mental clarity.

Core Fitness DVD – Focuses on effectively strengthening the abdominal muscles with the Pilates-based exercises using the Fitness Ball. The 60 minute DVD includes a 40 minute workout on the Fitness Ball, a mini workout that targets your weakest areas, and exercises that can be done at your desk while sitting on the ball.

Resources

RELATED WORKS

Releasing Emotional Patterns with Essential Oils
– by Carolyn L. Mein, D.C., Vision Ware Press. Clear deep-seated, emotional patterns permanently with quick and easy techniques.

Excitotoxins: The Taste That Kills –
– by Dr. Russell Blaylock, neurosurgeon, Health Press (1-800-643-2665).

Defense Against Alzheimer's
– by Dr. H.J. Roberts, diabetic specialist (1-800-814-9800).

For more information on aspartame:

- www.aspartamekills.com
- www.dorway.com

CONTACT INFORMATION

To order, or for additional information, contact your health care professional, nutritionist or local distributor. Or contact us directly.

Phone: (858) 756-3704

Fax: (858) 756-6933

Online: www.bodytype.com

Visit BodyType.com and click SHOP

Body Type Products

Books

Different Bodies, Different Diets™ — Women's Edition & Men's Edition. These two dietary and body typing guides are based on more than 20 years of research. The **25 Body Type System**™ was created to optimize health and vitality. Following the diet designed to support their body has allowed people who have tried diet after diet, with little success, to take off excess weight and keep it off. Actual photos of real-life people provide realistic pictures of what your body would look like if you were overweight, underweight, or at your ideal weight. This book allows readers to determine their body type and to then discover the specific diet most appropriate for them.

Different Bodies, Different Diets™ — Combined Edition. This edition published by HarperCollins contains photos of both men and women. Celebrities are referenced for each body type, along with one week sample menus.

Releasing Emotional Patterns with Essential Oils — A practical guide to the use of specific essential oils for clearing emotional patterns. It contains over 500 common emotions from "fear of abandonment" to "worry". Also included are charts showing the location of body alarm points, as well as reflex points on the hands and feet.

Additional Body Type Publications

Body Type Profiles and Diets - 25 Individual Booklets
Body Type Questionnaire - Men and Women
25 Body Type Photos - Men and Women
Microwaves & Dietary Myths
Advanced Dietary Guide
Body Type Essences
Muscle Testing

DVDs & CDs

Body Type Interviews (DVD) — Contains TV interviews of Dr. Mein on News 13 Los Angeles, New Attitudes, Inside Edition, KUSI News, Channel 10 News, KABC Los Angeles, KTLA Los Angeles and Southland Today. Ideal introduction to the body type system – great for patients and clients.

Core Fitness (DVD) — Focuses on effectively strengthening the abdominal muscles and pelvic floor with Pilates-based exercises using the Fitness-Fun-Ball™. Includes exercises you can do at your desk using the Fitness-Fun-Ball™ as a chair.

Chakra Harmony (DVD) — Harmonize your body, mind and spirit with essential oils and toning.

Body Type Training Seminar (CD) — Contains 6 CD's of live training seminar showing how to determine 25 different body types.

For Seminars, Lectures, Certification or Professionals in your Area

Call **(858) 756-3704** or visit our website at **www.bodytype.com**